MW01242824

PARKINSONS DISEASE

TRAPPED

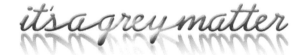

Christopher Evans

A modern day essay on the shaking palsy

Self published

All rights reserved. No part of this book may be reproduced or stored in an information retrieval system (other than for the purposes of review) without the express permission of the author in writing.

The right of Christopher Evans to be identified as author of this work has been asserted by him in accordance with the copyright, design and patents act 1988.

©2012 Christopher C Evans

This work is registered with the UK copyright service: Registration No:284660778

ISBN 13:978-1494241049
ISBN 10:1494241048

Typeset and Produced by www.clickcreate.biz, Iwade, Sittingbourne, Kent, United Kingdom.

Printed and bound in Great Britain by Orbital Print, Sittingbourne, Kent, United Kingdom.

Front cover image from istock.

Note: The material contained in this book is set out in good faith for general guidance and no liability can be accepted for loss or expense incurred as a result of relying on particular circumstances or statements made in this book. The laws and regulations are complex and liable to change and readers should check the current positions with the relevant authorities before making personal arrangements.

Where there is any suggestion in this book indicating types of medication that might be considered for testing, the author wishes to make it clear these treatment suggestions are for testing only and are NOT recommended for patients to experiment with. None of this information is to be used by patients as it has not yet been tested. This information remains theoretical for the analysis of the medical research profession and pharmaceutical testing only.

Acknowledgements

I cannot express enough gratitude to Graham Wallace; he has been instrumental in sculpting the scientific facts found in this book into a form suitable for non academics, a great challenge and very much an art, requiring great skill. Wallace is an expert in the art of English language and literature, and is a subject specialist in this work. His time and input have been invaluable. Thank you Graham, this book would never have materialised without you.

Jemma and David Rannard of www.clickcreate.biz have been fantastic. The cover design and illustrations throughout the book and website really complement the text. Professional, enthusiastic, efficient and always very helpful.

Particular thanks to my fiancée Michelle and the boys' for all their help, patients and understanding during this project.

John Moor, important mentor and good friend, appreciation for your guidance and feedback.

Joanne Davies, special thanks for proof-reading and feedback.

Kevin Ralph @ Images by Ralph, many thanks for design on the original brain diagram and book covers.

Other special thanks go to:-

Lynne Rye	Terence Moorcroft	Claire Lane
Mike Mein	Paul Ralph	Liz Orme
Lisa Payne	Dawn Hill	Dave Jupe

This book is dedicated to Lillian

Care, connect & cure those severely affected by Parkinson's disease.

The intention here is that this book will inspire:

- More directed and focused research leading to greater understanding.

- Advanced treatment and improved care.

- Earlier detection leading to better prevention.

- Increased awareness through accessibility.

New approach to Parkinson's disease

Christopher's modern day essay on the shaking palsy both questions and expands our understanding of Parkinson's disease. Accessible and meticulously researched, his observations illuminate the grey matter of brain science.

Evans' 20 years of clinical expertise and research skilfully brings together the latest facts on Parkinson's disease research. He examines three regions of the brain, the tasks performed by these regions and how they relate to symptoms of Parkinson's disease, highlighting insights that lead to the discovery of a unique potential cause.

Exploring the effects of trauma and lack of blood supply to the brain, he finds missing pieces to the Parkinson's puzzle.

This book:

- Explains why people, who smoke cigarettes, drink too much alcohol, are on blood pressure and cholesterol medication, and drink coffee excessively, are actually **less** likely to get Parkinson's disease.

- Looks deep into the art and science surrounding this contentious medical mystery.

- Introduces Evans' neurovascular hypothesis which explains new observations on vascular pathogenesis and brainstem primary involvement.

- Presents a controversial new three phase model of neurodegeneration which will challenge our current understanding of Parkinson's disease.

- Pushes boundaries of medical science and research in Parkinson's disease to a new level.

- Aims to *untrap, liberate or show a way* out for people suffering Parkinson's disease in the near future.

Contents

Preface

Imagine, for one moment, the horror of being trapped.

Most people can identify in some way with the feeling of being trapped. In Parkinson's disease there is a real sense of this. As degenerative brain changes take place, one inevitably loses mobility. Sufferers of Parkinson's may lose their jobs and fall into financial problems. The gradual loss of independence and control is significant and sufferers will have difficulties interacting with people and maintaining good relationships. This, alongside physical and emotional debilities, can have life- changing consequences. Some say it is like a second - somewhat surreal – life, because the life they have now is so different from the way things once were.

TRAP is an acronym readily used and understood by the medical research profession that describes four main symptoms of Parkinson's. It stands for: Tremor; Rigidity; Akinesia; and Postural instability. This acronym has been adapted slightly for the title adding: 'Parkinson's Education' (all together spelling the word 'Trapped').

The title *TRAPPED* works on many different levels. Parkinson's patients feel physically trapped within their own bodies. With inadequate medical treatment and fewer research opportunities in the future in the UK, it may seem that there is no release from this physiological entrapment. Hopefully, the work that follows will take treatment to the next level, the way out of Parkinson's.

Similar words to *trap* include: *confine, control, constrain, entrap, inhibit, lock-in, impede, imprison, restrict and obstruct.* Although these words are descriptive of how the

11

sufferer feels when Parkinson's strikes, they are also seen throughout this work; for example: 'specific arteries being *obstructed* which may *inhibit /impede/ restrict* blood supply to motor *control* centres in the brain leading to Parkinson's disease'. Antonyms for *trap* are: *release*, let go, *free*, *liberate*. This work hopes to liberate sufferers, from the physical *imprisonment* that is Parkinson's disease.

James Parkinson's writings were aimed to inform, teach and encourage further research. The work here has the same intention almost 200 years later. The use of complex scientific terminology has been avoided to make this work more accessible to those outside the medical profession and included is a glossary to help with any unfamiliar terms. Hopefully, the terminology will be understandable to all parties and the scientific research will be found interesting to non-academics. To this end, general education on Parkinson's has been included along with relevant scientific research.

Research will hopefully follow on from the suggestions made here and lead to a medical breakthrough.

Trapped has been in my mind for almost ten years. It was expected that someone in the scientific community would have similar ideas by now and thoroughly explored or tested them but this did not happen. So, I carried out my own exploration to see if missing pieces of the Parkinson's puzzle could be found.

With this new approach, I hope to connect with patients, groups, educational and pharmaceutical-organisations and disseminate this information to all interested parties including all experts in the field. I see this kind of cooperation similar to the way in which neurons interconnect and interact to facilitate information transfer between regions of the brain, joining forces for greater good of the body and brain, if one may use this analogy.

Some find accessibility an issue with any science as they are left with fragmented and isolated pieces of information. Others find articles in journals socio-phobic and disconnected from the people who have first hand experience of the diseases written about. Some find science ambiguous due to language misuse and snobbery meaning that even experts from different disciplines do not understand each other and what use is that?

A more ideal scenario would be a forum of experts from different disciplines not only talking to one another but also to patients. Imagine connecting researchers and experts from various backgrounds (for example vascular and neurological) working as a collaborative team, pooling resources, sharing information and together pushing the boundaries of known science in this field. This is the way forward and should, these days, be easily attained with use of internet social media.

The process of writing this modern-day essay on the 'shaking palsy' has taken considerable time and would, perhaps, have been much easier if my ambition had been restricted to producing a paper published in a scientific journal for self promotion. However, I chose, instead, to work with an expert in English language and literature to make this work as accessible as possible. I aimed for something that would not be found overwhelming and confusing but would be easily understood by as wide a range of people as possible.

Chapter One

Introduction & Overview

Introduction

Now is the time to focus on the subject of aging and degenerative brain diseases. We must develop treatment specific methods and neuroprotective pharmaceutical agents to prevent and target neurodegenerative disorders as we face increasing morbidity and rising care costs. This study will focus on Parkinson's disease: its nature, past present and new thinking on the cause, treatment and its imminent future potential.

Since early observations on this debilitating condition, there has been the drive to understand more of this and other degenerative brain diseases such as dementia. We are living in a world where the average lifespan is increasing. Needless to say, more funding is needed to help tackle the rise of inevitable neurodegenerative disorders. One study showed that in the last 100 years, there has been a massive increase in the population of elderly people (age 65 and older). Elderly people in the US made up only 4.1% of the population in 1900, but 8.1% in 1950 and 12.8% in 1995[1]. By 2050, it is postulated that 20% of the population will be 65 years old or older[2] (assuming people's health will continue along this line). Regarding this, newspaper journalists have been using phrases such as 'the dementia time-bomb'.

Speculation in science-fiction stories present ways in which the problem may be dealt with in the future. The novel In The Light of Other Days by Arthur C Clarke and Stephen Baxter, for example, suggests the use of 'cognitive enhancer studs' for the 'silvering of America'

---

[1] See Georgia Zachopoulos, *Current Trends in Health Care Costs* at http://www.case.edu/med/epidbio/mphp439/Health_Care_Costs.htm
[2] Ibid. See also: http ://faculty.washington.edu/chudler/aging.html

which stimulate 'the production of neurotransmitters and cell adhesion molecules'[3]. Fiction aside, the problem needs to be dealt with in reality and fast.

So, we see the imperative of finding ways to deal with this and where possible find a cure. Treatment of Parkinson's also needs to change. Looking at the treatment of symptoms is insufficient. So, attention must also be given to the greater question of the root cause where we may ultimately find this cure.

Modern technology has improved treatment and diagnoses. Computer games, apps and voice recognition technology on mobile phones are now helping Parkinson's sufferers[4]. With recent advances in diagnostic scanning technology, we may consider finding cures to be an effortless task. Yet, we cannot always rely solely on technology for the diagnosis and prevention of Parkinson's. Modern medicine's evolution has used scientific approach and innovation but, in reality, it is the skills of the clinicians and researchers and how they make use of the facilities that is of paramount importance; this is the real art. It is their knowledge that ultimately leads to cures. Technology doesn't ask the questions; it usually helps with the answers. It is man's ability to question that separates us from machines and it is this that is crucial to bring about solutions. In this process, we must use our vision, creativity and passion, along with logical and analytical thinking, if we are to progress to the next level of future health care.

---

[3] See page 50 of Arthur C Clarke & Stephen Baxter, *In The Light of Other Days* Voyager 2000

[4] Such as the iTrem which researchers hope will replace subjective tests in the assessment of tremors

Research is, of course, the key to all this. In my view, experienced clinicians should more often be encouraged to contribute to medical research to expedite answers to today's questions as it is through their wisdom and skills that we have the art of diagnosis. These are the people who are directly in touch with the patients and see more than just the physiological changes. As the patients deteriorate from a relatively healthy person, these practitioners will also see the affect on families and loved ones. This makes them experience the reality of their patients' condition in a far more direct way.

It is unsurprising that new theories on Parkinson's disease have not been forthcoming as it is an extremely challenging and complicated task to discover a cure. This study aims to explore the nature of cause rather than attempt to explain fully how we may be able to cure this condition. By understanding the cause we may find the cure as a result. If, on the other hand, a cure remains elusive, treatment can only be enhanced by a better understanding of the cause.

Often it is easy to underestimate the complex variables involved when finding a cure and researchers paradoxically obsess over these complexities. Here, it is my intention to keep things straightforward as simple ideas tend to be better than complex theories.

Current hypotheses on the mechanisms relating to Parkinson's disease need re-evaluation and new consideration should be given to alternative mechanisms which may reinforce or refute conventional ideas on the subject. My belief is that the present model is outdated. We must surpass old theories and reach a new understanding. As more recent studies show, Parkinson's is not solely a dopamine or movement disorder problem.

Current treatment is based on a model presented over 50 years ago, which may be one reason as to why treatment is focused around the motor symptoms and not the underlying cause. This is not unreasonable as, until now, there has been little success at reasoning an alternative hypothesis leading to greater understanding in the causation of Parkinson's disease.

This thinking and approach will prove controversial and it is my intention to challenge conventional thinking on Parkinson's disease. I make no attempts to be apologetic for any aspect of my neurovascular proposition that may prove disagreeable to the everyday academic attached to this area of study. Criticism is an essential part of scientific progress so we must constructively question and evaluate old concepts if we are to advance in any one particular field of medicine.

Future practice and treatment of Parkinson's may be changed in a positive way as result, directly or indirectly, of this work. I would also like to stress that I have been fortunate to this point, unlike many academics, to be free from the constraint of institutions that might otherwise drive this work in another direction or those likely to be motivated by profit, the 'curse of the vested interest'. I have conducted this work independently and there are no conflicts of interest, including any relationships with people or organizations that could inappropriately influence this study.

The aim, in what follows, is to introduce and explain the underlying principles and mechanisms involved in a new model which I have termed the Evan's Neurovascular Hypothesis and will also propose how and why this theory should be tested.

To this end, I will briefly outline current understanding primarily focused around the substantia nigra and its role in the production of dopamine which is (for now) at the epicentre of the neurodegenerative disorder we call Parkinson's disease. Specific pioneering techniques, methods and approaches will also be outlined and we will see how early diagnosis can be accomplished.

This work is not a comprehensive study on Parkinson's and some prior knowledge on the subject is assumed. Failing this, the reader may choose to undertake further research using the bibliography as a starting point. Salient points are needed to understand Parkinson's disease and the following text will refrain from detail one can easily find elsewhere as this area of research has been extensively covered. Stem cell and gene therapy are not covered; these are generic treatments, not specific to Parkinson's, and have been thoroughly researched over the last fifty years or so.

Instead, I have investigated alternative theories in pursuit of a single hypothesis explaining causative mechanisms in idiopathic Parkinson's, researching journals, books and various online resources. This has formed the basis for the science used as a foundation for my theory. I will be discussing relevant theories and studies with the intention of relating them to my own ideas and reinforcing them. Here, I have focused on abstracts and conclusions of current research and have integrated my own thinking.

This text will validate the new hypothesis regarding the cause and cure of this terrible affliction. Many books and papers I have read give an explanation on current thinking but I have seen few attempts at alternative detailed hypotheses on the causes of Parkinson's. I hope that these ideas will be considered and explored further.

Overview

The ideas presented in this book are based on functional neuroanatomy. This study may provide a potential breakthrough in the medical science of Parkinson's disease which may revolutionise treatment. It concerns the vertebral artery and how reduction in blood flow or ischemia can affect certain areas of the brain, how the brain is affected by reduced blood flow and what part the vertebral artery, in particular, plays. I will also discuss how specific symptoms of PD match those areas of the brain served by the vertebral artery.

I compare and simplify neuroanatomist Braak's 6-stage model into three phases but discard his viral pathogen theory in favour of a neurovascular hypothesis. In this model there are three main areas of targeted neurodegeneration of the brain. From this, we will see how the function of each area relates directly to Parkinson's symptoms. Rooting the progression of degeneration to these areas, we see that PD begins with brainstem ischemia due to reduced blood flow from vertebro-basilar artery degeneration or trauma.

Before exploring these ideas in detail, we will need to discuss the development of theories stemming from James Parkinson's initial observations as documented in his *Essay on the Shaking Palsy*. We also need to evaluate contemporary thinking on PD and treatment of the disease. Present day treatment is inadequate, making continued research into this territory and books such as this necessary.

There is a need for a new approach and a better way to treat those afflicted with the condition. Considerations on neurovascular activity form the basis of a hypothesis that may launch advancement in treatment. Once this has been established, clear suggestions are made on how treatment may be conducted in future and this is seen as being a long-term solution to problems with present-day treatment.

The text ends speculating on how this may be applied to similar neurodegenerative diseases and appeals to others that may join in future research to explore and fully develop this hypothesis.

Chapter Two

Grey Matter

Grey Matter

Any study of Parkinson's disease requires an understanding of how the brain operates. Today's thinking focuses on the part of the mid brain called the substantia nigra. We are still uncertain as to the origin of the problem and how PD develops in the first place. Looking at just one part of the picture, however, may restrict our sight to the degree that we are unable to locate the true origin of the problem. This is, at least, the impression I am left with after reading present literature on Parkinson's. The brain as a whole must be considered. We see, here, that any worthwhile study of neurodegenerative diseases requires us to observe brain regions in less isolation.

The true complexity of the human brain is presently beyond man's comprehension. We know a lot more now than we did fifty years ago about individual parts but we do not completely understand the brain or indeed how the mind works. However, we know it is extraordinarily interconnected. Some parts may appear to work independently but actually, communications between regions within the brain are intelligently and autonomously orchestrated. These regions of the brain function collectively for the continued existence of the whole organism.

Malfunction of any one region of the brain will therefore influence other areas, having internal and external effects. There are a number of ideas and theoretical models on how diseases such as Parkinson's progresses. The three-phase model discussed in detail later in this book, describes the disease process as following a kind of targeted serial pathway of neurodegeneration. In other words, the disease progresses through specific areas of the brain ('targeted' regions) and in a particular sequence (following a 'serial pathway'). This begins in the brain stem, working its way up through the mid brain and ends in cortical regions. These are wide ranging effects which are sequential in nature and can end in dementia.

The point here is that the brain is a complex system. So, looking at one part in isolation is not enough when considering any disease process (pathology) even if it can further our understanding. Exploration in any field of science inevitably draws attention to finer details but in doing this our view of the whole can be lost.

A good friend of mine (JWM), an expert in his field, explained computer systems in this way: "When we inspect the sub-systems in fine detail, we lose the effect those sub-systems have on the entire system and the effect the entire system has on the sub-system. Once we have a model of the entire system, it is easier to see the effect of changes in each direction." Treatment and pathological progression models of PD can also be seen in this sub-system way.

PD treatment is based on work undertaken a long time ago when our understanding of this condition was even more limited than it is today. There is a lack of understanding of the entire system which has been the barrier to treatment advancement especially when it comes to the limitations on the long term effectiveness of treatment.

As treatment is focused on the sub-system of movement and dopamine, we can now appreciate how and why this treatment has been limited. We are now aware of additional non-motor and non-dopamine sub-systems. This should enable new models of the entire system to become understandable, leading to treatment advancement of the entire system, rather than treating more sub-systems. This study aims to identify and present these new models of the entire system.

To begin with, let us view the brain as the organic structure that brings the mind into being. It is seen as operating on a primitive and instinctive reward-punishment system that primarily maintains our ability to adapt and survive in our environment. We have to control action to survive.

These actions include minute physiological adjustments. Maintenance of body functions - such as temperature, blood glucose and oxygen levels - is crucial for basic survival. This process of homeostasis is regulated through a collection of nuclei we call the hypothalamus. This also includes generating the circulation of chemical secretions we call hormones.

Action will of course involve - on a larger scale - voluntary rhythmic, synchronised motor actions (i.e. movement of limbs) and this is brought about by motor neurons. All control over these functions depends on – at a cellular level – neurons and their ability to release, receive and respond to neurotransmitters (essentially electro –chemical signals that will result in changes to other neurons or cells).

Neurotransmitters inevitably affect overall brain function. Some say our state of mind is determined by the biochemistry of our brains. Others argue the opposite whereby negative thoughts adversely affect brain chemistry. This gives us an *internal* versus *external* forces argument. Neither argument can be proved absolutely. Either way, we can not entirely separate mind from body. However, studies on the Placebo Effect[5] suggest a combination of the two models is more accurate.

The brain may be seen as a central hub or *hard drive* for signals or information being processed and relayed about our bodies and our environment. With such an analogy, it is easy for us to draw parallels with modern information technology. Indeed, some see the brain as an advanced organic computer, being a kind of 'intricate information exchange', albeit a complex one. We have even conducted virtual simulations on neural activity.

Despite this, there is much about the brain that eludes our understanding. The idea that our brains are like a biological computer is perhaps a little over-simplistic. Computers don't suffer neurosis, obsessions or psychosis. The computer, at best, can not enter into an exchange of dialogue in the intelligent way our brains can.

On a basic level, the brain receives and stores data in a similar way to a computer. However, it processes, interprets and modulates this information in ways not yet possible for computers, leading to complex patterns of data output for action, reaction or inaction. These interactions with one's environment make our brains unique. It can execute complex patterns of motor activity effortlessly - such as taking a cup of tea up the stairs in the morning - in a precise rhythmical, coordinated fashion.

Some will again draw comparisons between global communication and the way neurons interact, connect and

---

[5] See Brooks, Michael, *13 Things That Don't Make Sense: The Most Intriguing Scientific Mysteries of Out Time,* Profile Books, London 2010: Chapter 12: The Placebo Effect (p. 164-181); See also Chapter 1 of Hamilton, David, *It's The Thought That Counts: Why Mind Over Matter Really Does Work*, Hay House UK Ltd, 2008

communicate and help each other within the brain (such as the internet, Facebook, LinkedIn, Twitter and many others). Yet, it has also been said that the combination of every computer on the planet would not equate to the supremacy one human brain. The difference between the brain and a computer is that the brain has a mind of its own. We are gifted with consciousness which is seen as 'the controller'.

The study of artificial intelligence (AI) has become a discipline, focusing on providing solutions to real life problems. One of the biggest difficulties with AI is that of comprehension and self-awareness. Our brain's capacity for these qualities is remarkable.

So, we see that understanding how the brain operates is a complex affair. Its structure is also complex. Yet, it consists of three main regions. These three regions are the forebrain, midbrain and hindbrain. In the midbrain, we find the basal ganglia, and it is amongst this group of brain components that resides the substantia nigra (black substance) where dopamine is produced.

Dopamine is one of those neurotransmitters that play a part in the reward-punishment system mentioned earlier and it is this that has its role in addictions of one sort or another. It is also this neurotransmitter, or rather lack of it, which is the key consideration in the study of Parkinson's disease. We need to expand beyond our microscopic perspective in order to find new solutions.

31

Questions addressed throughout the book:

- How useful is the current knowledge on PD?
- Do we understand PD sufficiently to provide sufficient care to sufferers?
- Do we understand enough about the circumstances of how PD originates?
- If we do, is it possible to reduce the onset of PD?
- Why is the study of vascular pathogenesis affecting the brainstem important in Parkinson's?
- How are parts of the brain affected from a lack of nutrients resulting from a compromised blood supply?
- What is the role of brain stem function and how is it implicated in Parkinson's?
- What is the role of the basal ganglia function especially the substantia nigra and its significance to Parkinson's?
- Do current theories on Parkinson's help us treat this condition?
- What will advancements in Braak's theories achieve?

Chapter Three

Identifying Parkinson's

Identifying Parkinson's

Parkinson's disease is seen primarily as a movement disorder. A person suffering from the condition will suffer stiffness, increased muscle tone and postural instability with imbalance and a tendency to fall, slowness of movement, impaired dexterity, lack of facial expression, drooling and decreased blinking. Perhaps an easy symptom to identify is involuntary shaking which is more prominent when the sufferer is resting.

Other symptoms such as freezing, shuffling gait, stooped posture, small handwriting, insomnia and depression are also occasionally evident. Although this disease generally affects people over the age of 65, younger patients have been diagnosed with it also. Young-onset (for those affected under the age of 40) Parkinson's progresses more rapidly and is more difficult to treat.

An acronym used for Parkinson's symptoms, already mentioned in my preface, is TRAP. This stands for: Tremor; Rigidity; Akinesia; and Postural instability. 'Triad' is not an acronym but is often used to describe the three major symptoms of Parkinson's resting tremor, rigidity and bradykinesia (slowness of movement). This is more accurate than the akinesia in the acronym above as this is simply loss of movement. Bradykinesia is specifically slowness of movement which may involve difficulty in initiating movement.

Only two of these features are needed for the clinical diagnosis of Parkinson's and *true* diagnosis can only be ascertained after death via autopsy. The two pathological features are substantial loss of dopaminergic pigmented neurons in the substantia nigra and Lewy body inclusion in the remaining brainstem. However, Lewy bodies are a feature also found in other neurodegenerative disorders such as Alzheimer's so diagnosis of Parkinson's is even then uncertain.

Those afflicted by Parkinson's disease will undergo a drastic change in lifestyle and will experience isolation as they become fearful of others witnessing their symptoms. As the condition progresses, their activities will reduce making them prone to depression and loneliness.

Chapter 4

21st Century Parkinson's Treatment

21st Century Parkinson's Treatment

The science of medicine is being continuously updated with the use of research and new technology. What was a pioneering breakthrough 50 years ago, in the form of dopamine therapy, may now be outdated. New and exciting treatment modalities will be a revolution in the way we view and treat Parkinson's in the near future.

At present Parkinson's is treated by medical management and surgical management. Medical management is focussed on:-

1) Replace the missing dopamine

2) Block the breakdown of dopamine

3) Reduce the activity of acetylcholine

4) Introduce agents that mimic dopamine

5) Block excessive action of glutamate

6) Optimise delivery of levadopa (see **Figure 1**)

Figure 1

Medication used for Parkinson's

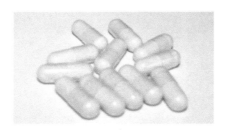

Sinemet Levadopa/Caridopa	Levadopa combined with carbidopa (helping the levadopa reach the brain). Initially works for most patients but has side effects of increased uncontrollable movement.
Comtan (Entacapone)	Used to help make the above work when its effectiveness starts to decrease
Dopamine Agonists - ropinorole/requip -pramipaxle	Stimulates the brain into making more dopamine. Less side-effects than levadopa and are more enduring. More suitable for younger patients but may tend to cause hallucinations and disorientation with more elderly patients.
Monoamine agonist - **selegiline** *(Eldepryl / Zelepar)* - **rasagiline** *(Azilect)*	Increases dopamine production but less commonly used. Fewer side effects than the above medications but dangerous to use with other drugs (eg. Antidepressants). Also may induce high blood pressure depending on diet.

Surgical management (mostly thalamotomy and pallidotomy) was phased out for a while when levadopa was introduced. However, more recently, surgical management has increased in popularity due, predominantly, to limitations of dopamine therapy and new advancements in scanning and surgical technology; we also have a greater understanding of basal ganglia circuitry.

An alternative to drug treatment, developed originally as a cardiac pacemaker, was adapted for Parkinson's patients, during the 1980's, in the form of deep brain stimulation. Deep Brain Stimulation (DBS) is a treatment modality involving surgery, used on patients who meet particular criteria. Electrodes are placed into the brain in the region of the sub-thalamic nuclei. These are then connected to a device similar to a cardiac pace maker which sends electrical impulses to stimulate dysfunctional areas of the brain. This is done with the patient conscious and requires patient cooperation throughout the operation so that precision in surgery can be millimetre perfect.

DBS (or less commonly known as an implantable pulse generator) results in increasing a patient's ability to move, thus reducing slowness of movement and easing the severity of muscle rigidity. It is also used to treat long term side effects of medication such as dyskinesia/ dystonia (i.e. abnormal, involuntary movements). The effects of deep brain stimulation on motor symptoms are extremely impressive. This becomes apparent when the patient turns off the device; instantly, the patient regresses to their pre-surgical state. The speed of this change is remarkable to see. It is being trialled in the treatment of depression and in other areas of medicine such as spinal injuries.

DBS is, however, a treatment that works only for some sufferers and not all. Furthermore, the procedure has cost implications and can give variable results. There may also be inconsistencies with long term use[6].

There are alternatives already emerging which may replace or coexist with deep brain stimulation. An implant exists which stimulates the spinal cord and may prove to be just as effective as deep brain stimulation. Another alternative is transcranial magnetic stimulation. This involves neural stimulation by electro-magnetic fields and is currently under development as far as PD treatment is concerned[7]. Advantages over DBS include the fact that these alternatives are both far less surgically invasive.

Dr Romulo Fuentes and colleagues from Duke University Medical Centre carried out the research. Their experiments on this device - in 2009 - showed previously immobile mice becoming active within seconds of the device being switched on[8]. This study explored effects of a low frequency current on nerves that run along the spine in mice (called Dorsal Column Stimulation or DCS). The mice had symptoms similar to PD, namely reduced movement. Electric current was delivered through

[6] See the Metro article: *Get a heads-up on the future with pioneering brain technologies* published Wednesday 24 April 2013 at

http://metro.co.uk/2013/04/24/get-a-heads-up-on-the-future-with-pioneering-brain-technologies-3664020/

[7] See Anon, *Transcranial Magnetic Stimulation for the Treatment of Parkinson's* Bio—Portfolio, August 2013 at:
http://www.bioportfolio.com/resources/trial/127230/Transcranial-Magnetic-Stimulation-for-the-Treatment-of-Parkinsons-Disease.html
Also see: http://clinicaltrials.gov/show/NCT00753519

[8] See Anon, *Spinal implant for Parkinson's* at:
http://www.nhs.uk/news/2009/03March/Pages/SpinalimplantandParkinsons.aspx

electrodes to nerves exiting the mice's spines, whilst the researchers observed the effects on their movement.

The study used a semi-invasive method to restore movement in two different PD models in mice. The research showed that DCS plus levadopa is superior to levadopa alone which could potentially complement existing treatments for early stage Parkinson's. The researchers hope to use primate models as these would more closely resemble how treatment might work in humans.

Although there is much promise in recent surgical management, we can not predict - at this stage - its long term effects. In the meantime, treatment of PD is mainly medicinal. We see here a kind of swing from one mode of treatment to the other as long-term effectiveness or side effects become apparent in both surgical and pharmaceutical treatment modalities.

There are presently problems associated with drug treatment of Parkinson's, mostly to do with decreasing effectiveness and adverse and unwanted effects. I have taken this list from the NHS website[9] and used it to create the following table (**Figure 2**).

---

[9] This list of side effects can be seen in full (as last revised in 2009) on the Clinical Knowledge Summaries (CKS) web site [http://www.cks.nhs.uk/parkinsons_disease] – date of observation: 27/09/2013

Figure 2

Physical Side Effects	Mental/Behavioural Side Effects
Nausea and vomiting Motor complications, including: Motor fluctuations. Dyskinesias Dystonic or akathisia-related pain. Daytime hypersomnolence or excessive drowsiness. Sleep disorders. Autonomic disturbances. Diarrhoea: May be caused by entacapone. Dose reduction may be needed. However, diarrhoea is sometimes severe enough to warrant discontinuation. Excessive saliva (sialorrhoea) Excessive sweating (hyperhidrosis). Hypotension: Tends to occur at the start of treatment with levodopa, dopamine agonists, and selegiline. Can usually be managed by dose reduction and slower dose escalation. Peripheral oedema: May occur with amantadine and dopamine agonists, but is not dose dependent. Diuretics or discontinuation of the offending medication may be considered. Postural (orthostatic) hypotension. Weight loss.	Neuropsychiatric symptoms, including: Cognitive impairment. Confusion and vivid dreaming (visual and auditory hallucinations): As with psychotic symptoms, these symptoms can be caused by dopamine agonists and (less commonly) levodopa, selegiline, and amantadine, and by any medicine with an antimuscarinic action, including some antidepressants and antipsychotics. The causative drug may need to be withdrawn. Impulse control and related disorders, including: Hypersexuality. Pathological gambling. Compulsive eating or buying. Punding — repetitive mechanical tasks, such as assembling or collecting. Dopamine dysregulation syndrome — compulsive dopaminergic drug use beyond that required for motor control. Psychotic symptoms.

As can be seen, this is an extensive but not unusual list of adverse effects and one could disapprove of them if there was an alternative. There is no alternative at this moment in time which is another reason why I have been encouraged to look at this problem from an alternative perspective. Present treatment is just not good enough.

As well as the classic symptoms, Parkinson's can bring about neuropsychiatric problems including disorders of: behaviour; mood; cognition and speech (see **Figure 3**). The severity of such disturbances varies widely.

Figure 3

Neuropsychiatric Symptoms	Description
Cognitive (Can occur in early stages or prior to diagnosis)	Problems with executive function (decision making, planning); initiating appropriate actions and inhibiting inappropriate Attention disorder Problems with learning and recall Visio-spatial difficulties
Mood and behavior	Anxiety; impulse control; depression; apathy; binge eating; medication overuse and craving
Body Function (Can occur in early stages or prior to diagnosis)	Drowsiness; insomnia; gastric dysmobility; visual changes; sensory changes (pain, numbness, pins and needles)
Dementia	Increased risk

At present, we understand the damaged substantia nigra to be the cause of motor symptoms but is this really the starting point, or do problems begin elsewhere? Perhaps the substantia nigra is merely part of a chain of events. To date, nobody has determined where Parkinson's begins but earlier non-motor symptoms may give us more of a clue as to the true origin of Parkinson's.

Next, we should also be questioning the idea that the substantia nigra is responsible for all Parkinson's symptoms. There are non-motor symptoms that are totally unrelated to this particular area of the brain. The authors of the book entitled Non Dopamine Lesions in Parkinson's Disease have also looked beyond the substantia nigra[10]. Here, one can find comprehensive writings on the subject of Parkinson's and I would recommend this (to academics) as further research which covers some of the issues I have reported upon in much greater detail. In the last forty years evidence of non- motor/non-dopamine symptoms such as Autonomic Nervous System (ANS) mood and sleep symptoms have been noticed and researched in greater detail.

It is clear that it is not enough to concentrate solely on the area of the substantia nigra and dopamine. For 21st Century treatment to progress, we need to look at a much wider picture as Parkinson's is multi-faceted. It is more than just a dopamine, movement or loco-"<u>motor</u>" disorder.

So, how, when and why did medical science become fixed on this notion that the substantia nigra and depleting dopamine is the focal point of Parkinson's? Was it because the motor or movement symptoms are the most easily identifiable? A patient's hands shaking uncontrollably or difficulties with their movement are the most visibly apparent and we see this as being the problem of primary significance. It is easy to see and, therefore, is the very thing we must fix. It is a visual world where evidence must be seen and 'seeing is believing' or was the introduction of dopamine responsible for this focus?

---

[10] See Glenda Halliday, Roger Barker and Dominic Rowe, *Non-Dopamine Lesions In Parkinson's Disease*, Oxford University Press 2011

It is easy to neglect those unseen problems that are as much a part of Parkinson's as movement difficulties. This would explain the overall fixation with movement mainly being the sole concern or 'target area' for treatment which may itself have rooted us from advancing further.

To get out of this trap of fixed thinking, it is useful to track how we got into it in the first place. Then, perhaps, the way out will seem clearer. The time has come to change the future by observing the past. In the next chapter we shall briefly look at the history of PD which will help to explain why things are focused around dopamine and movement.

Chapter Five

A Brief History

Parkinson Studies

James Parkinson was the first to study and write authoritatively about the condition which he called 'the shaking palsy'. Early descriptions exist dating as far back as the ancient world. However, many site Parkinson's work as the most significant starting point. His *Essay on the Shaking Palsy* was published nearly 200 years ago, in 1817. It was based on the cases of six patients, one of which he had examined himself. As with his other medical writings, Parkinson's style was not strictly detached in the usual scientific style, but mainly aimed to inform, teach and encourage further research. Since then, the ailment was identified as a medical condition and has been investigated more extensively.

Parkinson suggested that the origin of 'the shaking palsy' was from a diseased condition of the lower part of the brain from the high cervical cord through to the medulla. This is a remarkable deduction, despite limited knowledge of the brain in Parkinson's day as his ideas are not so far from current theories which place the substantia nigra as the main area of origin. Even so, Parkinson's suggestion regarding the origin of PD may be closer than we currently imagine as will be shown later.

Jean-Martin Charcot was the man who gave Parkinson's name to the disease and undertook further research. Looking for lesions in the brain, Charcot conducted autopsies on sufferers of Parkinson's. No lesions were found. This was to be discovered later. However, his studies on the disease, from 1868 to 1881, gave significant contributions to the work started by Parkinson.

In 1897, Brissaud, who understudied Charcot and rather ironically died of a brain tumour aged 57, interestingly Brissaud suggested that Parkinson's disease originated from ischemic damage.

Brissaud theorised that Parkinson's began in the region of the subthalamus or the cerebral peduncle from damage caused by blood deprivation (i.e. lesions resulting from ischemia).

Kustantin Tretiakoff, in 1919, identified the substantia nigra as being the part of the brain most damaged. With this, Triekiakoff led the way to modern thinking. However, it was not generally agreed that the substantia nigra was the region most affected until acceptance of Hassler's work. Hassler verified Tretiakoff's findings through his own research in 1938.

Arvid Carlsson's Nobel Prize winning work, in the 1950's, mainly provided the knowledge on the biochemical alterations and how the lack of the neurotransmitter dopamine brought on the motor symptoms of Parkinson's. His work on dopamine revealed the biochemical state of the brain activity of Parkinson's patients. This was to play a major role in modern-day treatment, which until then mainly involved brain surgery (from 1939). Now the drug, levadopa, synthesized by Funk in 1911, is prescribed as this is more effectual.

In more recent times, German anatomist, Heiko Braak, found those lesions in the brain that Charcot had suspected but failed to find. Braak began researching the central nervous system of fish. Further research focused on the patho-anatomy of the human nervous system; in particular: the cerebral cortex (in 1980).

He went on to research the neuropathology of Alzheimer's and later Parkinson's disease, classifying idiopathic Parkinson's into six distinct stages in 2003. Braak and colleagues advanced a 'dual-hit' hypothesis regarding the pathogenesis of Parkinson's to which an unknown pathogen, akin to a slow virus, may enter the nervous system through the nasal and intestinal mucosa resulting in a cascade of neuro-degenerative events affecting the brain.

A further contribution to current and generally accepted understanding of Parkinson's is the Frederic Lewy discovery, in 1912 of malformed proteins in affected brains (later to be called Lewy bodies).[11]

So, we have around 200 years of focussed study on Parkinson's disease. Yet, it seems that since the introduction of dopamine, we have not witnessed any major breakthrough in the treatment of PD. It seems that research has not really gone beyond the mid brain and this may be the reasons significant advancement has not been made. Looking back prior to the 50's, we see that areas of the brain stem were seen as worthy areas of investigation. This appears to have been abandoned since the discovery of dopamine loss in the substantia nigra. Yet, it is the brain stem that is worthy of review.

---

[11] See *What Lewy Body Disease Is* from The Lewy Body Journal at: http://www.lewybodyjournal.org/whatlbdis.html

Brissaud's theory of damage caused by blood deprivation is something that I am going to explore more thoroughly in the rest of the book. From this point the true cause of Parkinson's may have been overlooked and the emphasis of research on PD has been too fixed by mostly focussing on the one area.

Chapter Six

Modern Perception

Modern Perception

We know PD patients lack dopamine, a neuro-transmitter found in the brain. Dopamine is responsible for movement and it is the reduction of dopamine which leads to symptoms of Parkinson's. Dopamine is primarily manufactured in an area of the brain called the ventral pars compacta, part of the substantia nigra (black substance). It is thought that this is the primary area affected by Parkinson's disease. For reasons not yet understood, when 60-80% of dopamine is lost, symptoms such as slowness of movement, tremor and imbalance occur and this often results in the diagnosis of Parkinson's.

Although this problem with dopamine reduction is a problem in Parkinson's, it would be a misconception to assume that the malfunction of the ventral pars compacta is the cause of the disease. We can only be sure that it is a consequence of contracting PD.

Dopamine is also instrumental in reinforcing behavior and learning, certain stimuli activate dopaminergic neurons particularly those associated with reward, e.g. sex and eating, also in the substantia nigra, where dopamine is manufactured; there are types of neurons partly responsible for forming addictions. So there is more going on here than just movement attributed to this 'dopamine factory'.

A lack of dopamine will inevitably result in problems with movement and other brain functions. However, this is not the only problem. There are a myriad of non-motor symptoms that have been ignored up until recently. It is now well known that non dopamine (non motor) lesions precede the onset of motor symptoms[12].

Researchers have yet to determine reasons why the substantia nigra stops producing dopamine. As already mentioned, we can not really say that the cause of Parkinson's is a dysfunction within the substantia nigra and peri-thalamic structures. If medical scientific practice proved this area was central to Parkinson's disease, then modern day treatment would all but eradicate this disease. However, treatment targeting the substantia nigra has, so far, proved limited with variable results. L-dopa medications used to raise dopamine levels ultimately reduce the body's own ability to produce dopamine naturally and in time the receptors these substances activate are shut down, reducing the medications' effectiveness.

As we can see, this medication does not treat all the symptoms, nor is it neuroprotective as progressive degenerative changes continue to occur despite treatment. Keeping all this in mind, it is clear that this target area of the substantia nigra needs to be reconsidered. Other target areas such as the brain stem structures could be determined. Then the treatment of PD can take better aim and reach these new targets giving longer term benefits.

Currently we treat depleting dopamine levels. The main treatment 'bullet' of today is dopamine but this has led to the neglect of treating non-motor symptoms. So, there is a need to consider new models such as the one proposed in Chapter 8 which has the potential to cover not only motor symptoms but more likely the whole symptomatic picture

[12] See Halliday, Barker & Rowe (editors), *Non-Dopamine Lesions in Parkinson's Disease*, Oxford University Press, 2011.

of Parkinson's. It seems that since the introduction of levadopa, which was a fantastic breakthrough, there has been a general apathy to investigate new ground despite there being millions spent on research development. By new ground I mean to challenge the fundamental principles and theories that define Parkinson's disease. It would appear that few challenge these old models (Braak et al excluded). Yet, these models are used to form the basis of a lot of current research.

We need to know and understand the root cause of this dysfunction. Later, we will see more reasons why the substantia nigra is not the epicentre of Parkinson's. Chapter 8 gives a model which explains the evolution or pathogenesis starting in the brain stem leading to the mid-brain and finally to the cortex.

The role of non motor symptoms has nothing much to do with the substantia nigra and I use this to support a strong argument that the origin of Parkinson's is from structures elsewhere. The substantia nigra can no longer be seen as the main cerebral structure of origin when evidence now indicates the contrary.

It is time to change our old beliefs as these are decades out of date. We must agree on an alternative as the current focus on the substantia nigra and depleted dopamine production can only be a part (although an important part) of a greater picture. The pharmaceutical industry has a vested interest here and will eventually benefit from information found in this book; more important to me is the benefit this will bring to patients. This however, will mean embracing and investing in this new science.

Before discussing Braak theory, an understanding of the basal ganglia is needed. This is a very complex area. Instead of detailing the intricate regional interconnections, a diagram has been provided so that the models of circuitry are easier to interpret (see **Figure 4**).

Figure 4

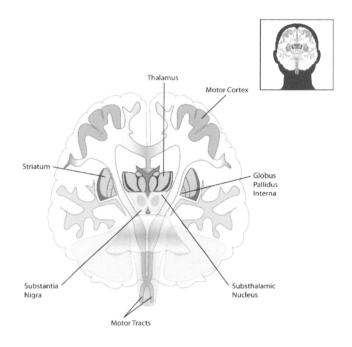

The basal ganglia, a collection of brain nuclei involved in controlling movement, includes: the caudate nucleus; the putamen; the globus pallidus; the subthalamic nucleus and the substantia nigra. Controlling movement is, of course, an essential function of the entire nervous system. It is the basal ganglia and, more especially, the striatum that are fundamental for instigating movement by modulation of motor neuron activity. Effective future treatment, for those suffering movement disorders, requires us to have a greater understanding of the movement process. For this, we would need to observe regional brain activity and how this relates to execution of movement.

The assistant Professor of Physiology and Neurology at the University of California, Anatol Kreitzer, acknowledges that we still have much to understand in this regard. He claims that a 'thorough knowledge of the mechanisms underlying circuit function in the basal ganglia, both in health and disease, will provide a framework that can be used to develop novel treatments for neurological disorders'[13].

Disease of the basal ganglia results in movement disorders. Movement disorders are characterized by hypokinesia (reduction of intentional movement) and/or hyperkinesia (uncontrollable involuntary movements such as tremor and writhing). Basal ganglia diseases include diseases such as Parkinson's disease (hypokinetic) and Huntington's disease (hyperkinetic). However, not all movement disorders result from dysfunction of the basal ganglia.

The basal ganglia play a significant role in Parkinson's disease, which involves degeneration of the substantia nigra. Huntington's disease primarily involves damage to the striatum. Basal ganglia dysfunction is thought to control other disorders of behavior such as the Tourette's syndrome, obsessive–compulsive disorder etc. The mechanisms underlying diseases of the basal ganglia such as Parkinson's and Huntington's are not totally understood and scientists are still developing theories on movement disorders.

Parkinson's disease and Huntington's disease symptoms are virtually polar opposites; Parkinson's disease is characterized by gradual loss of the ability to initiate movement, whereas Huntington's disease is characterized

---

[13] See: http://www.gladstone.ucsf.edu/gladstone/site/kreitzer/

by an inability to prevent parts of the body from moving unintentionally. These difficulties with initiating and controlling movement are among the most important symptoms.

As one problem is *hypo*kinetic and the other is of a *hyper*kinetic nature, it must be possible to treat Parkinson's by stimulating the Huntington's area of the striatum. Conversely, Huntington's could be treated by stimulating the substantia nigra. This idea is indeed being explored and exploited with great benefit for patients.

Deep brain stimulation is used in the treatment of both; specifically, the globus palidus interna (which is in the Huntington's area of the striatum) is targeted for the treatment of Parkinson's, and the subthalamic nucleus (which is just above the Parkinson's substantia nigra area) is used for the treatment of Huntington's. One can see in the diagram that these structures are in close proximity to the motor tract; therefore, it is not difficult to imagine their inhibitory or modulating effect on movement.

One research team, led by a Professor Redgrave[14], conducted a project that found destruction of areas of the basal ganglia (responsible for habits) can have a beneficial effect on Parkinson's disease. Professor Redgrave and his team propose that removal (surgically) of inhibitory output areas from habitual control circuits could make it easier for goal-directed behavior to be expressed. Inhibiting an inhibitory pathway results in exciting brain signals.

---

[14] See: *Research brings cure for Parkinson's disease a step closer* e! Science News.mht for article published: Tuesday, October 19, 2010 - 10:37 in *Health & Medicine)* @ http://www.shef.ac.uk/news/nr/1772-1.174113

The blood supply to the basal ganglia comes from the middle cerebral artery. Interestingly, Dr Peter Jannetta, in 2011, claimed to have cured a Parkinson patient by repositioning the posterior cerebral artery[15]. Some symptoms returned a week or so after surgery so the surgeon decided to operate on the side of the brain that was not treated. At the time of the report, Dr Jannetta was looking for Parkinson's patients to volunteer to help further this study.

The procedure mentioned above, called microvascular decompression (MVD), seemed to alleviate Parkinson's symptoms in the patient operated on. A detailed article on this, written by Jannetta and his team,[16] has been published in the *Neurology International* journal and raises some relevant questions: 'Can MVD relieve parkinsonism? Is there a form of parkinsonism related to arterial compression of the cerebral peduncle? Is Parkinson's disease in young people the same etiologically as in the older population? Are Cognitive changes reversible? Will MVD of the cerebral peduncle be as safe and effective as MVD is for other problems?'[17]

Narrow vessels in the area of the middle cerebral artery are a frequent site of cerebral haemorrhage in patients with uncontrolled hypertension. Small infarcts produced occlusion of these small vessels and are called lacunes. These may be asymptomatic and are discovered

---

[15] This artery is below the middle cerebral artery but they have a close proximity, the former having supply from the carotids; the latter will have supply from the vertebrobasilar arteries.
[16] See Peter J Jannetta, Donald M. Whiting, Lynn H Fletcher, Joseph K Hobbs, Jon Brillman, Matthew Quigley, Melanie Fukui, Robert Williams *Parkinson's disease: an inquiry into the etiology and treatment*; Neurology International Vol 3, No 2
2011[http://www.pagepress.org/journals/index.php/ni/article/view/2567]
[17] ibid

incidentally at autopsy or on MRI. However, lacunar[18] in the basal ganglia is thought to be linked to movement disorders (no doubt from functional anatomy of the basal ganglia).

I speculate that a similar link could be attributed to the posterior cerebral artery and the arterial branches below as they both branch from the vertebrobasilar arteries. This, as can be seen, will not have a direct effect on movement, but may lead us to understand the non-dopamine symptoms of Parkinson's (i.e. those not directly related to movement).

It is clear that the basal ganglia have a central role in motor control. They are also involved in learning and motivation. I have shown ways in which the blood supply is important. I would now like to look at other mechanisms which may have influence over the immobility of Parkinson's patients.

Management Strategies

Parkinsonian patients sometimes show a phenomenon (called *kinesia paradoxa*) in which a generally immobile person reacts to an emergency in a coordinated and mobile way, then, once the emergency has passed, lapses back into immobility. Thus motivation and other complex inhibitory control circuits and feedback mechanisms are slowly becoming more understood, although not fully. As far as I am aware, the mechanisms of this apparently paradoxical circuitry are, to date, unknown.

Exploiting the phenomena of kinesia paradoxa by utilizing visual and auditory cues has proved an effective

---

[18] *Lucunar* is Latin for *lake*. *Lucunes* is the plural form.

management strategy for a number of Parkinson's patients suffering movement disorders. These cues encourage focused movement and through their use, patients are able to greatly improve stride length and fluidity. One study has shown the use of visual cues enables movement for those who suffer lack of mobility (akinesia)[19].

Visual cues may take the form of lines on the floor or contrasting floor tiles. Special glasses, called virtual cueing spectacles, have been designed which visually project lines on the floor at the wearer's feet. These glasses are a more permanent and efficient stimulus and would work in most situations. Unfortunately, at this time, they are expensive.

Auditory cues are based on timing and rhythm. A book entitled Musicophilia by the famous neurologist Oliver Sacks has a chapter specific to Parkinson's. This fascinating book goes into detail of how music can affect normal brains including numerous other neurological disorders.

Of course, these audio and visual cues work in such a way as to help focus attention. Indeed, it has been found that patients may overcome akinesia to some extent by focusing on specific movements without visual or auditory cues of any kind.

An obvious advantage to this kind of approach is that it does not involve invasive brain surgery which may result in unforeseen complications, nor does it require the use of drugs which are likely to lose their effect or bring about

---

[19] Kaminsky, T. A., Dudgeon, B. J., Billingsley, F. F., Mitchell, P. H., & Weghorst, S. J. (2007). Virtual cues and functional mobility of people with Parkinson's disease: A single-subject pilot study. Journal of Rehabilitation Research & Development, 44(3), 437-448.

undesired side effects after a period of time. However, these visual and/or auditory cues have to be present for the treatment to work as once they are removed the patient's problems return. Furthermore, kinesia paraoxa is less likely to work for those patients in the more advanced stages of Parkinson's.

Researchers are attempting to explain the mechanisms of kinesia paradoxa by a defining theory. Understanding this phenomenon is of great importance. The solution to this puzzle would make a great advancement for scientific knowledge on the pathology of Parkinson's disease.

There is an interconnection between the limbic system and the basal ganglia. The limbic system - which has a role in emotion and behaviour, or as I have heard it called, the 'sex, drugs and rock and roll centre' of the brain - also affects the substantia nigral/striatal areas.

The limbic system, especially the ventral pallidum, the ventral tegmental and the nucleus accumbens (which are involved in motivation driven by addiction and pleasure/reward), is somehow stimulated by a conscious mental reflex releasing the neurotransmitter dopamine. The function of these areas and their interconnection, is becoming more understood and although may be confusing for those without knowledge of neuro-anatomy, they are fundamental for understanding the mechanisms of Parkinson's in more detail.

Chapter Seven

Braak

Braak's Viral Pathogen Theory and his Six Stage Model

Heiko Braak, as mentioned previously, classified idiopathic Parkinson's into six distinct stages which chart the pathological progression of Parkinson's. This will be further explored here to pave the way for the Evan's Neurovascular Hypothesis.

Underlying the pathology of Parkinson's is gradual brain degeneration. So, in studying the disease's progression, researchers look for damage in various stages. Using staining techniques, Braak found deposits of abnormal proteins in particular regions of those whose brains were affected by PD and dementia.

Cell death in the substantia nigra is a characteristic finding in Parkinson's especially the ventral area of the pars compacta. By the time a patient dies, 70% of dopamine-producing cells in these areas are dead or damaged[20]. These damaged neurons are thought to be caused by abnormal brain proteins called alpha-synuclein. Accumulation of the protein alpha-synuclein is found in combination with ubiquitin. These types of protein accumulate forming clumps known as Lewy bodies which become the identifying marker for neurodegenerative pathologies, especially Lewy body dementia (LBD) and PD. They are also thought to spread throughout brain matter causing irreversible lesions.

---

[20] Both Parkinsons.org and the Movement Disorder Virtual University state 70% of these cells die before PD symptoms become apparent. See http://www.parkinsons.org.au/about-ps/whatps.html and http://www.mdvu.org/library/pediatric/bradykinesia/bra_mec.asp

Degeneration of nigro-striatal axons is linked to the genesis of Parkinson's disease, in which degeneration of cell bodies leads to reduced pigmentation of the substantia nigra and subsequent reduction of dopamine. We currently understand this to be the process by which pathological changes lead to Parkinson's symptoms.

Braak's stages 1-6 postulates the progression of Parkinson's disease based on histological findings which lead to pathological changes. He identified Lewy body deposits in certain areas of the brain and that these progressed from the brainstem to the substantia nigra and cortical regions. He concluded that brain-stem damage was likely to be the first recognizable phase of Parkinson's. Further to this, it has been indicated that there is a significant reduction in the size and mass of the brain in a sufferer of Parkinson's disease in the latter stages.

Braak's six stages work as follows:

Figure 5

Stage 1	***Preclinical*** -Possible abnormalities of the autonomic nervous system, dorsal motor nucleus of the vagus nerve and in the anterior olfactory structures and medulla oblongata -Patients display few symptoms perhaps those related to autonomic function such as bowel motility and blood pressure changes.
Stage 2	***Preclinical*** -Abnormalities of the medulla oblongata, olfactory bulb, lower raphe nuclei and locus coeruleus -Patients display appetite and mood changes, depression, spontaneous pain, REM sleep disorder and attention deficits
Stage 3	***Possibly clinical*** -Lewy body cell changes in the substantia nigra, amygdala, mid-brain and basal forebrain -Patients may present with difficulty of movement, wondering attention, REM sleep disorder, sleepiness in the day, difficulty with thought processes involving planning and decision making; again, problems with depression
Stage 4	***Clinical*** -Neurodegeneration and Lewy bodies in the substantia nigra, gray matter nuclei midbrain, basal forebrain and temporal mesocortex -Obvious Parkinson's motor symptoms, behavioral changes and implications again of sleep disorder. Changes in the pedunculopontine nucleus
Stage 5	***Clinical*** -Lewy bodies progress to the amygdala, temporal neocortex, sensory and premotor areas. -Strong emotional changes are occasionally evident along with motivational difficulties
Stage 6	***Clinical*** -Lewy bodies may progress to the neocortex, cortex, and primary sensory and motor areas -Parkinson's disease dementia (different from Lewy Body demetia) may be evident along with any or all of the above

Braak and his colleagues proposed that Lewy bodies may be present a long time before diagnosis, and accumulation of Lewy bodies can be found in more distant areas than that of the substantia nigra, affecting neurotransmitters other than dopamine[21]. This suggests a lengthy preclinical phase of pathological degeneration.

Pathological progression studies suggest that there is a 7 to 8 year period between Braak stage 1 (during which there will be few apparent symptoms) to Braak stage 3 (when symptoms become apparent).

Braak's findings on the pathological progression of PD are, for me, still more significant than the discovery of the depletion of dopamine in the substantia nigra or indeed the discovery of alpha synuclien abnormalities (with Lewy bodies).

We must question why these abnormalities are present, what causes them and whether they are of significance. On post-mortem, a number of aged persons who had not been diagnosed with Parkinson's were found to have alpha synuclien abnormalities (with Lewy bodies). This has led many to disregard Braak's ideas and neglect their inferences.

You can find alpha-synuclein at post-mortem in *normal* individuals (i.e. those to whom neurological signs were not found) and this is why it has been said that there is no

---

[21] Some studies propose a pre-diagnostic non-motor symptom period of 5-20 years from the onset of PD to actual motor-symptoms (see Savica R, Rocca WA, Ahlskog JE, *When does Parkinson disease start?* Archives of neurology 67:798-801, 2010). For a study on PD diagnosis, see Lingor, Liman, Kallenberg, Sahlmann and Bähr, *Diagnosis and Differential Diagnosis of Parkinson's Disease* @http://cdn.intechopen.com/pdfs/20327/InTech-Diagnosis_and_differential_diagnosis_of_parkinson_s_disease.pdf

relation between Braak Staging and Parkinson's disease. In other words, detection of alpha-synuclein or Lewy body proteins is not a reliable indication of Parkinson's disease. Presumably, the human subjects autopsied in which "incidental" (of little consequence) Lewy bodies were found, had not ever suffered Parkinson's. However, it may be that, as with so many people, diagnosis of Parkinson's had not yet been ascertained. There is a difference between saying 'there is nothing to be found' and 'there was nothing found'. The former suggests there is nothing to be found at all, whereas, the latter statement does not rule out the possibility of something being there but was just simply not discovered.

One study found that structural, degenerative changes to the brain did not necessarily mean that neurodegenerative symptoms would follow, which was surprising. The Nun Study of Aging and Alzheimer's disease was founded by Dr David Snowdon to ascertain factors bringing about neurodegenerative diseases and began in 1986. The study of a group of Roman Catholic sisters of The School of Notre Dame was deemed advantageous because the sisters did not take drugs and drank little or no alcohol which would otherwise bring other factors (extraneous variables) into consideration.

Although the study is still ongoing, there have been significant findings. From examining texts written by the nuns, researchers found that those with high literacy skills were less likely to suffer Alzheimer's in later years. Around eighty percent of those whose writing lacked fluency, complexity and a wide vocabulary, developed Alzheimer's in old age whilst only 10% of those who were very able writers ended up with the same condition. The study suggests that there is a relationship between lack of cognitive abilities and susceptibility to neurodegenerative diseases[22]. This implies the benefit of keeping mentally active and gives credence to the saying 'use it or lose it'[23].

The overall significance of this study showed that a reduction in brain mass was no absolute indication of Alzheimer's or similar conditions. Structural brain changes observed in these subjects would, perhaps, lead to the assumption of a general mental decline. However, this was not the case.

In old age, some suffer mental decline while others do not. Factors other than brain mass must be making the difference. Surely, the brain's ability to adapt is a factor making these differences, particularly when the individual is mentally and occasionally physically active. Of course, it is well known that when someone is physically and mentally active, the circulation of blood to the brain increases, maybe this is another significant factor here.

This goes to show that there is still a way to go in our understanding of the brain overall. We are progressively increasing our knowledge of individual areas of the brain; but how these areas interact and interconnect with each other is something we are still exploring.

Relating brain mass to Alzheimer's seemed a logical idea but, as the Nun Study showed, was far from reliable. What seems obvious may, in the end, be doubtful. A similar case is found with the idea that Lewy bodies should correspond Braak staging.

---

[22] **See** The University of Minnesota's Nun Study FAQ page, 18 Dec 2009, http://www.healthstudies.umn.edu/nunstudy/faq.jsp

[23] A Science Daily article (dated March 6, 2013) reports scientific evidence to support the idea that a stimulating physical and mental activity protects against Altzeimer's.
See: http://www.sciencedaily.com/releases/2013/03/130306134224.htm

Braak's hypothesis that Parkinson's begins in the medulla, the enteric nervous system and the olfactory bulb, is supported by the non-motor symptoms evident in the early stages of the disease. This has led researchers to pursue ways of halting the progression of its pathology.

As already explained, Braak suggested a staged sequence of events. From the study of brains (post-mortem), it was concluded by Cambridgeshire and Nottingham researchers[24] (studying Braak's staging) that alpha-synucleinopathy is frequently associated with Alzheimer's. Nevertheless, a significant proportion of brains showed Lewy bodies in cortical regions and 29% were found to be amygdala predominant.

These latter findings did not correspond to Braak staging and this was unexpected. Basically, the study proved that incidental alpha-synuclein can be a found in aged people regardless of neurodegenerative pathologies. Therefore, in the study of neurodegenerative pathology, alpha-synuclein may not now carry as much weight as we once thought and perhaps it is now time to take a fresh perspective.

Braak staging suggests that Lewy bodies form first in the two main brain stem structures (the medulla oblongata and pontine tegmentum). At this time, overt symptoms for Parkinson's have not manifested. Nevertheless, Lewy bodies reach the substantia nigra as the condition progresses. Then, the disease reaches other areas, such as

---

[24] See *Patterns and Stages of α-synucleinopathy: **Relevance in a Population-based Cohort*** by J. Zaccai, PhD, C. Brayne, PhD, I. McKeith, MD, F. Matthews, PhD and P. G. Ince, MD at http://www.neurology.org/content/70/13/1042.abstract

the mid and forebrain and finally the area of the neo-cortex.

I have shown Braak's six stages in the aforementioned table (**Figure 5**) as this indicates, for me, a progression of the disease originating from brain stem to cortex. This should give the reader a greater insight into the theory I wish to present.

Although I refer to Braak repeatedly in order to substantiate and strengthen my own theory and to give the reader a comparative understanding so that one can visualise my own observations, Braak found changes initially in the olfactory bulb (during stages 1 and 2). I find the olfactory area a mystery and the viral pathogen supposition a difficult concept to accept.

It seems unreasonable that this disease process should start in two opposing areas (i.e. 'top': olfactory and 'bottom': brain stem) especially when the rest of Braak staging follows a sequential and logical order moving progressively upwards (superiorly) from the lower (inferior) brain stem structures through to the cortical or higher centres. Furthermore, smell loss may not necessarily be a non-motor symptom specific to Parkinson's but merely be a factor of normal ageing as Doty, Hawkes and Berendse note in *Olfactory Dysfunction in Parkinson's*, 'approximately half the population between the ages of 65 and 80 years and nearly three quarters of those over the age of 80 experience measurable smell loss' [25].

---

[25] See Halliday, Barker & Rowe (editors), *Non-Dopamine Lesions in Parkinson's Disease*, Oxford University Press, 2011, p.65 (Chapter 4).

It has, however, in more recent years, become accepted that visual and olfactory sensory changes are present in Parkinson's but the cause of the failing olfactory areas is still unknown. Although protein fragments of synuclein have been found within olfactory neurons, no one, so far, has discovered synuclein or Lewy body deposits in the nasal olfactory epithelium which should have shown early signs or elevated concentrations.

As to why Braak staging should start in the olfactory area simultaneously to the brain stem and how they connect is, at present, unknown. This warrants further investigation.

Braak conceived his viral pathogen theory by seeing a link between his Lewy body findings in the olfactory area and the onset of Parkinson's. One could also speculate that Braak's theories may have come about by matching PD symptoms with corresponding areas of the brain, after cross-examining the chronological pattern of symptom distribution. This may have led logically to the construction of his staging and creation of his viral pathogen hypotheses. Or to simplify, as one can see, there is a link between functions of the brain stem and Parkinson's non-motor symptoms. (See **Figure 6**).

Braak may have made, as I have, a connection between brain stem dysfunction and symptoms in Parkinson's which would have led him to deduce that Lewy bodies would also be found in Parkinson's disease as it is found in Lewy body dementia. He may then have tried to advance this concept by speculating his viral pathogen theory to which he sought validity through Lewy body findings.

Before researching Braak Theory, I had drawn a rough copy of the illustration (**Figure 6**) which directly connects

81

PD symptoms to regional brain activity, matching regional brain function with dysfunction in PD. I saw this connection between brain dysfunction and PD symptoms in 3 pathological phases[26]. I studied the functional anatomy of brainstem regions, as this is the area supplied by the vertebral artery. From this, I found there was a significant relationship between the function of the pons and the non-motor symptoms of Parkinson's (see **Figure 6**). This, one would imagine, Braak would have seen in his own studies.

Braak's theory and viral pathogen hypothesis has been welcomed but such an idea infers that PD is something you can catch, like a cold, only with more devastating consequences. To say that PD is something one can catch would not sit well with some researchers and academics in the field. The fact that Braak employs the medical terminology of 'a viral pathogen' makes the idea more palatable and apparently worthy of consideration. To say one can 'catch PD' does not nearly have the same ring even though it is saying much the same thing. It is certainly not something I can easily accept especially where he suggests PD starts as a "slow virus".

Nevertheless, credence has been given to the idea of 'catching' PD by some researchers and practitioners outside of Braak. Studies have been conducted on a group or 'cluster' of cases of people contracting PD who work closely.

Dr Donald Calne, of the University of British Columbia Hospital treats two of three cast members of the 70's Canadian sitcom Leo and Me who contracted the disease.

---

[26] However, unlike Braak, I have not the facilities available to me to study human brain tissue immunohistologically.

He claimed to the Chigago Sun Times that 'studies have found there to be an increased risk of clusters among certain workers who operate closely together.'

The scientific director and chief executive of the Parkinson's Institute in California, Dr J.W. Langston, is not convinced, and has pointed out that while some studies show this to be a possibility, others do not. He says, "You can find studies that people who spend time with each other are more susceptible to Parkinson's disease and you can find the reverse", and believes we are a long way to finding the cause of PD.

Another point to consider is that were PD to be caused by a viral pathogen, then close family members of PD sufferers would more likely catch the disease. Clearly, there is no evidence to support this.

PD is more likely to be a result of certain external factors that may be environmental and/or physical. I am inclined towards the idea that one may have a predisposition in combination with these factors. This could be genetic or as a consequence of a lifestyle-choice or even a long-term effect from an injury. All this will become clearer later when I will discuss my own theory.

Figure 6

How Parkinson's Symptoms Relate to Regions of the Brain

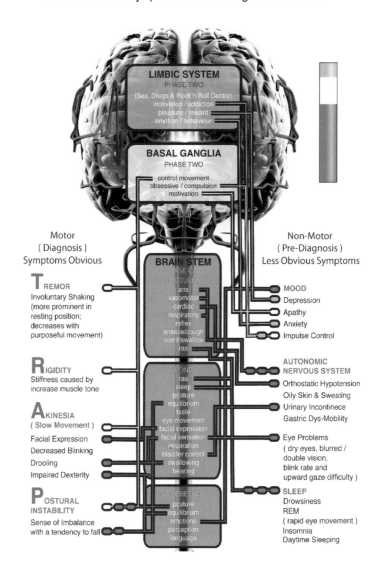

Figure 7

Symptoms

Medulla	Pons	Cerebellum
Ans	Sleep	Posture
Vasomotor	Posture	Equilibrium
Cardiac	Equilibrium	Emotions
Respiratory	Taste	Perception
Reflex	Eye movement	language
Sneeze/cough	Facial expression	
Vomit/swallow	Facial sensation	
	Respiration	
	Bladder control	
	Swallowing	
	Hearing	

Figure 8

Motor

Symptoms

(Post-diagnosis)

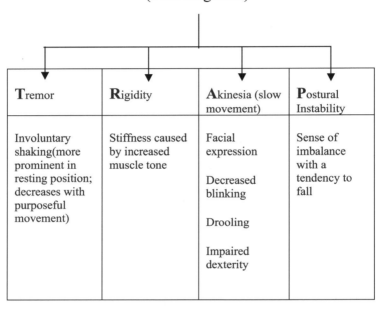

Tremor	Rigidity	Akinesia (slow movement)	Postural Instability
Involuntary shaking(more prominent in resting position; decreases with purposeful movement)	Stiffness caused by increased muscle tone	Facial expression Decreased blinking Drooling Impaired dexterity	Sense of imbalance with a tendency to fall

Figure 9

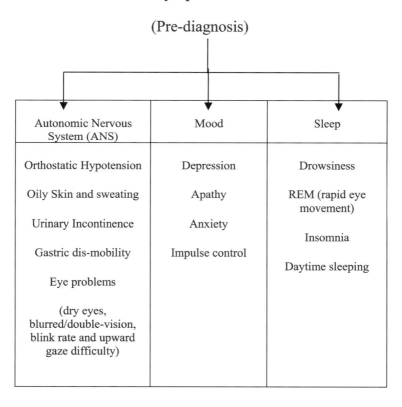

Non-motor

Symptomless

(Pre-diagnosis)

Autonomic Nervous System (ANS)	Mood	Sleep
Orthostatic Hypotension	Depression	Drowsiness
Oily Skin and sweating	Apathy	REM (rapid eye movement)
Urinary Incontinence	Anxiety	Insomnia
Gastric dis-mobility	Impulse control	Daytime sleeping
Eye problems		
(dry eyes, blurred/double-vision, blink rate and upward gaze difficulty)		

So, were Braak's results influenced consciously or subconsciously by his understanding of functional neuroanatomy? The results from the above tables (Braak's work **Figure 5**) match my diagram (**Figure 6**) almost identically except the olfactory area. Nevertheless, to achieve similar conclusions from two very separate methods of approach is astounding. That said, Braak's theories have been retested many times and the consensus is that they are to be generally accepted.

Let us assume Braak's staging is on the whole accurate. His insight and staging model gives a great foundation to work from and adds substantial weight to the neurovascular hypothesis presented later which may provide a number of missing pieces to this PD puzzle.

I have covered Braak's theory so that my ideas are more easily understood. We now also have a point of reference with which to draw a comparison. I hope the neurovascular hypothesis I present may go on to have a greater likelihood of acceptability and accuracy than Braak's viral pathogen hypothesis. However, I will let you, the reader, evaluate the following and decide for yourself.

I will attempt to show why, in Chapter 9, the neurovascular hypothesis and the neuro-structure/function model have the ability to mature into a theory.

Chapter Eight

Formulating a New Hypothesis

Formulation of the Evan's Neurovascular Hypothesis

My initial idea for what would become my neurovascular hypothesis originated in the late 1990's. At the time, I was treating Patient X for mobility problems. Patient X was the first of my patients to have Parkinson's. After dealing with more Parkinson's sufferers, I began to notice something other than the typical symptoms associated with Parkinson's. What I noticed, in common with these patients, led me to further study this interesting area of medicine. This theoretical insight sparked my curiosity.

This consistent finding was the loss of neck movement with a tendency for the head and neck to be positioned forward (anterior to the lateral centre of gravity line). This, one may argue, will simply be due to common C5/6[27] degenerative changes or the postural changes normally associated with PD. However, my view, at that time, was that the accessory nerve (CN XI), in addition to other lower brainstem centres, led to postural changes in this area. This is due to the motor accessory nerve affecting the resting tone of the trapezius and sternocleidomastiod muscles. So, the anterior head and neck position is fixed depending on favourable or unfavourable circumstances involving the vertebral arteries.

I considered that this may be an attempt of the body, in some way, to correct or adapt to a compromise in blood flow to the brainstem via the vertebral artery.

The other possibility is that the positional changes of the head and neck are, perhaps, as a consequence of accessory

---

[27] By C5/6, I mean the fifth and sixth cervical vertebra

nerve dysfunction, again due to a reduction of blood supply from the vertebral arteries. In other words, positional changes in the neck happen to relieve pressure on the vertebral artery which in turn affects the accessory nerve or simply they are brought about as a result of reduced accessory nerve innervation. Both scenarios involve a problem with the blood supply from the vertebral artery.

This idea of a reduced blood flow to the brain from the vertebral artery led to the formulation of my theory. Some elements of the theory were to change as time went by but ultimately the underlying basis of the theory with regard to the vertebral artery remains the same.

I would encourage the reader to research the function and location of the vagus nerve, it sits next to the accessory nerve and has been implicated by some as a possible cause of non motor symptoms in PD. This makes interesting reading and relates directly to information presented in this book.

All these ideas came about around the time I had the great fortune of meeting Patient X in the late 1990s. This was early in my career which was to be a very steep learning curve as I was at this time inexperienced in this area. Before long I gained more experience with many more patients with PD and similar conditions (50 or so patients).

Patient X was in some denial regarding the label/diagnosis of Parkinson's and refused to take prescription medication, despite having almost textbook symptoms and signs. There was an internal struggle with acceptance and a strong element of resistance. Confronting this diagnosis required putting a strategy in place, one that involved a battle of mind, will and self to overcome the obstacles, adversity and inherent suffering of PD.

Before retirement, patient X was a teacher and naturally taught me a lot about Parkinson's disease. It was a joy working with such a motivated and intelligent person. I very much admired and encouraged/supported this strong spirited approach.

Family history was somewhat repeating itself as X's mother also had Parkinson's. Chapters of X's life were opened to me each and every visit. The most poignant and illustrative detail was that X suffered repeated punches in the face as both a child and an adult. This really shocked me at the time and I still struggle to comprehend it now. To be able to help other extraordinary people like this was the incentive behind these writings.

Previous to my contact with Patient X, I had studied in some detail the anatomy of the vertebral artery along with clinical consequences related to this area such as vertebrobasilar insufficiency and the test for this (VBI). So, a depletion of blood supply to the brain stem via the vertebral artery immediately jumped out at me as a possible causative factor. The only person I knew (prior to Patient X) that had Parkinson's was the great Mohamed Ali; therefore, trauma to head and neck was the link made at the time.

For a long time, I was not able or inclined to study this further as I was researching the mechanisms and treatment of stress. So, research in the area of Parkinson's involving complex areas such as the brain would have to wait. Thus, 10 years or more passed until this conundrum became a persistent pre-occupation that simply could not be ignored. Finally I listened to what my mind was telling me and put pen to paper.

Chapter Nine

The Evans Neurovascular Hypothesis

The Evans Neurovascular Hypothesis
Figure 10

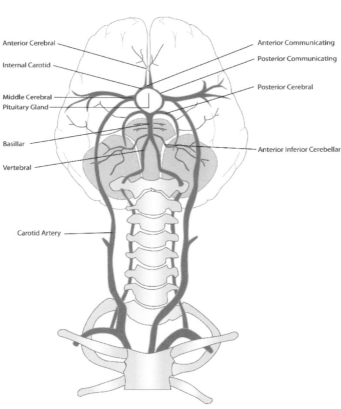

Anterior Cerebral

Internal Carotid

Middle Cerebral
Pituitary Gland

Basillar

Vertebral

Carotid Artery

Anterior Communicating

Posterior Communicating

Posterior Cerebral

Anterior Inferior Cerebellar

In the diagram (**Figure 10**) one can see the clear anatomical relationship between the vertebral arteries and the brain stem structures.

The vertebral artery is crucial to the brain stem function as it supplies blood, fluids and nutrients to these structures. The brain stem structures are of primary importance in Parkinson's so we must investigate how this process of supplying blood is crucial to optimal brain function. Only then may we ascertain the origin of Parkinson's and hopefully reverse the condition in its initial stages.

The brain stem area is the starting point from which a cascade of events unfolds prior to the secondary area of the substantia nigra (currently accepted as the primary 'brain centre' for Parkinson's disease).

I propose ischemia[28] via the vertebral-basilar arteries to be a root cause of idiopathic Parkinson's disease from either internal or external mechanisms/forces. Also, I suggest that immunohistological changes, such as Lewy bodies etc., may be a consequence of these ischemic changes. This may be why Lewy bodies can be found in people that do not go on to display clinical signs of Parkinson's. You may feel this is a bold statement as why Lewy bodies form in the first place and what defines them is still uncertain and a matter of speculation.

Hypothetically, ischemia in the vertebral artery presents three possibilities: one will lead to the onset of idiopathic Parkinson's with Lewy bodies present; another ends with Lewy body dementia with or without PD present and the third possibility is the apparent absence of either one of

---

[28]Ischemia is the condition of diminished blood flow and supply to a detrimental extent.

these two. Nevertheless, given this last outcome, structural neurodegenerative changes still occur but may not lead to the patient displaying obvious symptoms, like those in the nun's study. A normal elderly person, for example, who may be difficult to classify, will elude a diagnosis due to an uncertain clinical picture. Only meticulous research will establish the exact sequence (stemming from ischemia) that leads to any one of these three possibilities.

Looking at the diagrams (**Figure 6** and **Figure 10**) again, we clearly see an anatomical connection between the vertebral artery and brain stem structures. We can also see the interrelationship between structure function and symptoms.

It is accepted within the medical profession that damage to the mid-brain from major vascular causes is likely to result in PD. Conventionally, vascular PD (sometimes termed 'multi-infarct' Parkinson's) strikes suddenly. A vascular cause is usually by an obstruction or bleed (as in brain haemorrhage). Rapid cell death follows. This is not how I suggest neurodegenerative changes in idiopathic Parkinson's take place at all. Few, if any, to my knowledge, have considered the idea that slow micro-vascular changes could indeed result in the onset of progressive idiopathic Parkinson's symptoms. Furthermore, no one to my knowledge has looked extensively at the vertebral artery as being a principal underlying or primary factor. So, it is a known fact that vascular mechanisms can bring on 'vascular' Parkinson's. How is it, then, that slow ischemic micro-vascular changes to the vertebro-basilar artery, as I propose, have not been thought about seriously or even previously considered?

A research team led by Aron Buchman (from Rush University in the USA) found that blocked blood vessels in the brain may be implicated in Parkinson's. These micro-vascular arteriosclerotic changes are often too small to be seen with standard medical imaging techniques. However, the team reported that these blockages were significant and are associated with changes in gait which were similar to those seen in Parkinson's. This has led to the thinking that such blockages may be involved in Parkinson's pathology[29]. The team urged for 'more aggressive prevention and treatment strategies for vascular risk factors.'[30] Although they found micro-vascular changes, they do not seem to have specified where the problem begins, nor have they determined what regions of the brain are affected by these vascular changes. These findings fit my neurovascular model but the study conducted by the Buchman team differs. They merely imply these micro-vascular changes are part of the disease process, whereas I see dysfunctional vascular mechanisms as being the root cause. Nevertheless, their findings and my theory have common ground; both indicate neurodegeneration from micro-vascular changes occurring in arteries supplying the brain.

It seems to me more likely that ischemia over time brings on gradual, subtle and eventually observable signs of Parkinson's.

---

[29] See *Brain Blood Vessel Blockages May Contribute to Parkinson's Disease* by Aron S. Buchman, Sue E. Leurgans, Sukriti Nag, David A. Bennett, Julie A. Schneider. [http://www.worldhealth.net/news/brain-blood-vessel-blockages-may-contribute-parkin/]

(Posted Sep 25 2011)

[30] ibid

The neurovascular hypothesis suggests idiopathic PD is caused by micro-vascular ischemia due to A) internal factors (weaknesses and predispositions) and the effect this has, is dependant on, or influenced by B) external factors (physical, chemical and mental traumas) in combination or alone which directly correlate to susceptibility or inevitability of disease onset.

So, two groups form the basis of the theory.
These are:

  A. Internal mechanisms. (Susceptibility)
  B. External mechanisms. (Inevitability)
These can be further broken down into two groups.

These are:

  A1. Arteriosclerosis
  A2. Reduced cardiac output, diabetes, nutrition, exercise, stress etc;
  B1. Degenerative/postural changes (i.e. cervical spondylosis /osteoarthritis)
  B2. External factors post traumatic (i.e. physical/mental/chemical trauma.) viral/post encephalitic, post traumatic stress, alcohol, drugs prescribed and non-prescribed etc.

In the case of (A1), the diameter of the arteries diminishes preventing adequate blood flow. This is caused by degenerative changes common around the age of onset of Parkinson's by a build up of plaque in the lumen of the artery resulting from damage and/or an increase in cholesterol deposits.

(A2) - Reduced cardiac output combined with narrowing of the vertebral artery - may be of significant importance and I have devised an equation considering these important factors so that this may be more thoroughly tested. This could also be applied to diabetes and other factors which may ultimately influence blood flow to the brain stem structures.

(B1) - Degenerative cervical spine - The vertebral artery passes through narrow foramina in the transverse process of each vertebra, six through to one, entering the scull through the foramen-magnum. The narrow foramina through which the vertebral artery passes can be obstructed by either positional changes of the vertebra (i.e. osteoarthritis) or osteophytic encroachment brought about by normal wear and tear, genetic predisposition or whiplash type effects to the cervical spine. Compression of the vertebrobasilar artery is also possible as the artery passes through the foramen-magnum and thereafter.

I suggest that (B2) post-traumatic cause i.e. physical/mental trauma. Physical traumatic causes can be from early childhood through to adulthood. The long-term effects of brain injury from concussive and sub-concussive head trauma have been studied. Some studies conducted in this area initially assumed that head trauma preceded Parkinson's; researchers thought that this was not the case. Conversely, it was concluded that symptoms of imbalance had led to the trauma. Nevertheless, this data was considered just prior to the onset of symptoms of Parkinson's.

Further enquiry into traumatic causation from 15 years back or more was not pursued as is with patients suffering dementia pugilistica. It is my belief that we would benefit from a more extensive medical history of Parkinson's patients with relation to physical trauma. Physical trauma is an area needing focussed research. This is where I would be inclined to start searching as recent research seems to indicate strong associational links.

Mental stress/trauma, such as is seen in post traumatic stress disorder patients, is a very interesting area. The focus of this book does not allow me to elaborate here. Suffice to say, certain sights, sounds, smells etc can have a triggering physiological effect on brain chemistry and function thereafter, ultimately leading to structural brain changes. Incredible as it may seem, this is a real possibility as mental trauma can on occasion be more devastating and longer lasting than physical trauma. Shell-shock (combat stress reaction, posttraumatic stress disorder, post-concussion syndrome), for example, can have a powerful effect, involving chemical/physiological changes in the brain. Stress is a subject I have studied in great detail which can render a victim catatonic. I recommend consulting material by Oliver Sachs (such as his book/film, Awakenings) for discussion on similar research findings into encephalitis lethargica. Researched material, which links to chemical trauma, is also readily available. Combinations of the above are likely to increase ones propensity to idiopathic PD.

I have discussed external and internal mechanisms and why these increase one's chance of Parkinson's and other neurological diseases later in life. I have shown examples of research on how optimising blood flow to the brain makes a positive difference in treatment of Parkinson's and this ultimately has to do with restoring blood flow and cellular repair. Now I would like to look at what happens at this cellular level and give examples of impact scenarios to illustrate how variables affect an individual's case.

Ischemic Damage:
How Lack of Blood Affects the Brain

Ischemia is brought about by lack of adequate blood supply. There is not enough blood to supply the required oxygen to tissue. Tissues require oxygen to produce the energy used to maintain and repair cells.

If these cells are starved of oxygen over a certain period of time, they will suffer irreparable damage. Brain and heart cells, for example, can be irreversibly damaged in as little as three minutes. Cell death occurs in these tissues leading to brain or heart damage. There is also a 'cascade' process of damage to the tissue involving a build up of metabolic waste substances (excretes) and the inability to maintain cell membranes which results in a leakage of unwanted enzymes into those cells compromised[31]. This is the general picture of ischemic damage. It may occur for any organ of the body. The brain is no exception.

There are two types of ischemia in the brain[32], (sometimes called 'cerebral ischemia'). One is focal – occurring in a specific region of the brain – and the other is global which is wide-spread throughout the brain. Both involve obstruction and haemorrhaging. As focal ischemia affects a specific area, it is clear that this threatens any particular part of the brain local to that area. Cell death will occur and so tissue damage follows.

---

[31] For more information on ischemic cascade, see Hinkle JL, Bowman L. "Neuroprotection for ischemic stroke". *J Neurosci Nurs* **35** (2) April 2003
[32] See Lipton, Peter, *Ischemic Cell Death in Brain Neurons* in Physiological Review Vol. 79, No. 4, October 1999 (Printed in the USA)

It may initially seem that a resolution to the situation is to restore normal blood flow as soon as possible. But, the problem here is that an immediate restoration of full blood flow will not redeem the situation. In fact, it can make matters worse and this is called reperfusion. The reintroduction of oxygen in the system brings with it damaging free radicals and an increase of calcium which will - in effect - accelerate cell death. There is also the problem of white blood cells absorbing damaged cells which left alone may survive.

Having said all this, there is still the fact that the brain is able to recover from global ischemia if blood supply is restored within a certain time frame - not too fast and not too slow. Furthermore, the use of vasodilatory drugs results in a gradual widening of blood vessels. If blood supply is restored gradually, problems of reperfusion must surely be reduced. Again, time factor has to be an absolute consideration. There is a window of time in which to reverse ischemia and save the threatened area of the brain and this must also be a gradual process of restoration.

Sudden or acute cell death is, of course, an adequate explanation for vascular PD but this is not the case for idiopathic Parkinson's disease where the onset is slow and insidious. Evidence would be easily identifiable from an MRI scan seen when liquefied cells form a cist-type structure but this is not the case, PD is not visible on MRI.

When cells have been starved of oxygen and have not liquefied, they maintain their basic structure but are dead, nevertheless. So, could the ghost-like appearance of cells be an indicator of idiopathic PD as this shows a slow or chronic cell-death process? Only after death and under microscope, could this be used as a starting point, but would obviously be of little value to the dead patient diagnostically. As again this will not show on MRI.

The name substantia nigra (Latin for 'black substance' as one might recall) was given as this is part of the brain that is dark in colour. As dopaminergic neurons are lost here this black pigment melanin lightens. Could this change of colour be the effect of the accumulation of our 'ghost-like' cells that have died due to ischemia rather than the reduction of melanin or a possible combination of both?

Linking Impact Brain Damage with Ischemia

In the February 2011 edition of the National Geographic (unconventional reference material granted), there is an interesting article on chronic traumatic encephalopathy (CTE) affecting American football players who sustained repetitive head blows (protective helmets worn) linking CTE with Alzheimer's. There is an image comparison between three brains: a normal brain, a (CTE) and an Alzheimer's brain, giving a representation of micro and macroscopic changes. The macroscopic images of the CTE brain and Alzheimer's brain show obvious physical similarities in brain stem and cortex. Comparing all three brains, the CTE brain appears to be somewhere between the healthy brain and the Alzheimer's in terms of deterioration. It is as if the CTE is part of the progression towards Alzheimer's.

Investigating brain swelling (of those American football players who have worn helmets) would perhaps be of primary interest. However, we already know this to be an issue from other sporting injuries including dementia pugilistica from sub-concussive blows. I would be more inclined to include changes to the cervical spine in my investigations as these lead to arterial and slow ischemic brain changes.

I am linking ischemia to head blows because when tissues suffer impact they swell. The swelling of any tissue will put pressure on neighbouring structures. In the brain this is particularly significant as the skull is a force resisting pressure and as fluid is incompressible, the brain structure will be the target of this compression. Blood vessels within the brain will be compressed especially those towards the cranial base or brain stem. As hydrostatic pressure builds, there will be a force felt from above. The vessels below will have constrained blood flow. The result will be cellular ischemia leading to cell death.

Famous Cases

With boxers such as Mohammed Ali (Cassius Clay)[33], it is obvious that sub-concussive blows are likely to lead to brain damage[34]. Other famous PD sufferers talk of brain trauma, including the brilliant anatomist Gunther von Hagens[35].

Despite a great understanding of the human body it remains uncertain if Gunther himself would make any association between his brain trauma and his PD (although it seems to have had a significant "impact" on his

---

[33] Around 15-20% of Professional boxers are said to get Dementia Pugilistica which involves Parkinson's syndrome
(see: http://www.dementia.org/types/dementia-pugilistica).
[34] See Freidman JH, *Progressive Parkinsonism in Boxers*, Pub Med US Library of Medicine 1989 (found
@http://www.ncbi.nlm.nih.gov/pubmed/2655100)
[35] Journalist Russell Working informs us that when Gunther von Hagens "was 6, he suffered a nearly fatal head injury and spent 11 months in the hospital" and at "one point a physician told the boy he was going to die." See
https://sites.google.com/site/stopbodyworlds/media-coverage/russell-working

childhood memories from this time). He unfortunately suffered a near fatal head injury as a young boy, decades prior to the onset of his own PD condition[36]. He, as well as many others, would no doubt rule out any suggestion that his trauma and his PD are linked due to the enormous time lapse of around 50 years or so, which would be considered tenuous.

Ali appeared to develop PD like symptoms within a far shorter time frame than Hagens so why would the onset of PD for one person arrive more slowly than another? Some may see huge incongruity concerning these two cases. However, despite this discrepancy in time and circumstance, I nevertheless see they may be strongly related for many reasons.

In medicine you can not simply apply the same scientific and mathematical principles to human pathology that you can apply to other scientific disciplines. As said before, there are too many complex variables to consider. This is a point made in the book, *Describing a Rose with a Ruler* by Nic Rowley. The title alone reminds us that human beings, like roses, are individual and unique. Let us use the example of Ali and Hagens to illustrate why things are rarely text-book in medicine.

As young Gunther was a haemophiliac, any head injury would have resulted in an increased chance of bleeding and subsequent raised intracranial pressure leading to possible ischemia as described above. This would have caused significant neural damage at the time.

---

[36] Von Hagens acknowledged he had Parkinson's in 2011 (See: *Exhibitor of Bodies Intends to Contribute His Own*, New York Times, published 5 January 2011).

A child, however, can be more resilient and has a greater capacity to recover from head trauma than an adult due the greater capacity for neuroplasticity. Ali, on the other hand, was an adult when he sustained blows from boxing, which were recurrent and sub-concussive. Conversely, Gunther's head injury was a single event trauma where severity, susceptibility and age are some of the variables which must be taken into account.

Usually, however, there is even more to consider. Parkinson's is not a condition we can precisely diagnose[37] , especially when it comes to determining an exact starting point. As we have seen, it is only when people show motor symptoms that they tend to be diagnosed. They cease to be seen as normal and become patients labelled with a disease.

Hagens may have been suffering the initial phase of PD many years before he began experiencing motor-symptoms. With many physical traumas, the effects can be delayed until old age. One can, for example, be predisposed to osteoarthritis from either a single major event trauma often decades prior to its onset or, conversely, from decades of minor micro-trauma such as repetitive strain analogous to Ali.

Ali's onset in 1984, three years after his retirement, may not be as quick as we think especially when we consider that he had a 20 year career. From the 60s to 1980, he was notorious for not being knocked out (good for boxing but not for the brain). He also had just over 100 amateur

---

[37] On the basis of clinical observations, PD diagnosis is 75–80% accurate. See Jankovic J, *Parkinson's disease: clinical features and diagnosis, J. Neurol. Neurosurg. Psychiatr.* 79, April 2008

bouts. His symptoms were noticed before 1984 but were misdiagnosed as a thyroid disorder[38].

Ali and Hagens had more than just head trauma and PD in common. Both personalities were compulsively driven, which may indicate early non-motor symptoms way before their diagnosis of PD. This may have been the force behind their successful careers, which begs the question of just how long these people had suffered PD completely unaware.

Neurodegeneration and Ischemia

There is a simple reason why I suggest cerebral ischemia from vertebral artery insufficiency to be integral to the origin of idiopathic Parkinson's. The principle may even apply to other neurodegenerative diseases (especially dementia). All the cells in the body, including neuronal cells, need adequate and plentiful blood supply for growth and repair. The blood contains essential nutrients for the health and sustainability of cells. Therefore, if a cell is deprived of blood supply its function will be affected and its very existence threatened.

We can see that cells that are lacking nutrients will have impaired function. There is a mathematical relationship here, an inverse correlation between two variables; as blood, nutrients and oxygen decrease so the rate of degenerative changes will increase proportionately, due to cell death.

Let us examine the concept of degeneration. It may be described as gradual deterioration of specific tissues or

---

[38] For a biography on Mohammad Ali, see Hauser, Thomas *Muhammad Ali: His Life and Times*, Robson Books 2004.

cell replication with impairment of function, caused by trauma, disease, aging or the immune system turning against self. Cell degeneration occurs more as we age or it may, in fact, be better to say cell regeneration occurs more slowly as we age. We may see, here, a direct link between blood supply and cell regeneration.

So, what may appear to be a degenerative condition is in fact due to a lack of the body's ability to regenerate cells fast enough to facilitate complete cellular repair. Degeneration then, almost anywhere in the body is an illusion that has resulted from this apparent lack of timely or complete cell regeneration, not, paradoxically, an increase in degeneration. This is important to understand when we view neurodegenerative disorders. Cells have not simply started to degenerate or die; they have always done so from the beginning and continue to degenerate/die at a relative equivalent rate. However, it is the regeneration process that slows or malfunctions in some way as we age. One perception is that cell degeneration acts as a destructive, external force. Conversely, I see it as a consequence of the body's internal repair system slowing (or being impeded) but no longer able to keep up the rate of maintenance required, death being the ultimate example.

The delicate balance of degeneration versus regeneration is crucial for health. In this way neurodegenerative disorders may actually be seen as disorders of neuro*re*generation. The big question for me and you is *why?*

The exact cause for nigral cell loss is still unknown[39]. Could a deprivation of blood supplied from the vertebral artery lead to eventual compromise of cell regeneration in the substantia nigra region which in turn results in an inability to produce dopamine leading to motor symptoms clearly evident in Parkinson's patients? Similarly, could, non-motor symptoms (and this is of greater importance) again result from the above same failing blood supply of the vertebral artery which leads to compromised cell regeneration affecting brain stem structures, which takes place some years earlier to the diagnosis of Parkinson's easily identifiable motor symptoms.

A logical and sequential order to view this disorder would be working backwards from symptoms of Parkinson's, looking at the relationship between function of the brain and PD symptoms, then observe those regions which may be affected. From the development of these ideas I deduce the following:-

Brain stem structures are the missing link to our understanding of the cause of idiopathic Parkinson's. Crucially, the reason why this is so is that the vertebral artery provides these brain stem structures with an adequate blood supply. The brain stem consists of three important areas: the medulla oblongata, the pons and the cerebellum. The function of these structures is of paramount importance if we are to further our understanding of Parkinson's.

---

[39] See *Dopanimergic Neurons* by Chinta and Anderson in The International Journal of Biochemistry and Cell Biology, May 2005

The functions of these structures are as follows:-

The medulla oblongata is responsible for the functioning of the autonomic nervous system which includes: the vasomotor and cardiac centres, respiratory centres and reflex mechanisms of sneezing, coughing, vomiting and swallowing.

The pons function primarily deals with sleep, posture, equilibrium, taste, eye movement, facial expressions, facial sensation, respiration, bladder control, swallowing, and hearing.

The cerebellum mainly controls posture and equilibrium. Aside from this, it regulates emotions such as fear, depression, happiness and euphoria as well as being involved in cognitive functions such as perception and language.

On observation of the function of the pons, medulla and cerebellum, one notices that a direct link clearly exists between Parkinson's symptoms and the dysfunction of the brainstem structures. (See the following diagram – **Figure 11**).

Symptoms are discussed in Chapter One.

Figure 11

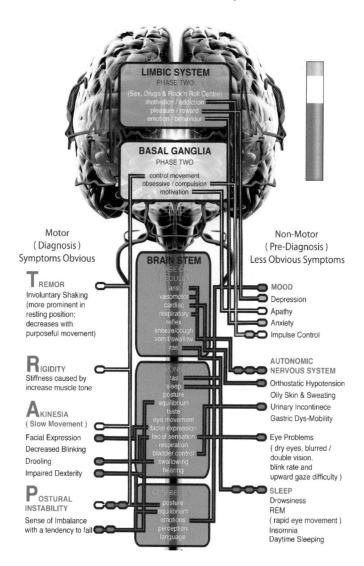

How Parkinson's Symptoms Relate to Regions of the Brain

On closer inspection of the above diagram, we see that there is an inter-relationship between functions of the pons and some Parkinson's symptoms. Some may argue that most of the symptoms associated with this area are not significant so we should disregard the pons as a target area of interest. However, this is an area of the diagram **(Figure 11)** that has the most interconnecting arrows. Clearly, there is a connection between the pons and PD symptoms. The pons can not be disregarded that easily when studying Parkinson's and the diagram makes this apparent.

So, we have a set of symptoms, related to the pons, that are present often years prior to diagnosis. At this stage, Parkinson's diagnosis is difficult to ascertain. It is when motor symptoms become more evident that a diagnosis is made. This is synonymous with Braak's Staging Theory. The positioning of the vertebro-basilar arteries is, I believe, of great consequence and is not merely coincidence. The implication of this suggests that Parkinson's disease may manifest itself in the pons area, the medulla and possibly the cerebellum thus bringing about these early symptoms. Later the disease will progress superiorly targeting the substantia-nigra which leads to the more obvious and easily identifiable Parkinson's motor symptoms.

Until more recent decades, researchers and clinicians were only looking at these dopamine based motor-function symptoms and in doing so have disregarded the possibility that Parkinson's may begin elsewhere such as in the pons region or lower brainstem centres. Knowing the history, we see this is similar to what James Parkinson, Brissaud and latterly Braak asserted.

The Evan's Tri-Phase Model

I have reworked Braak's 6 stages, simplifying them into 3 phases. The resulting tri-phase model is in chronological order:

Phase 1: subthalamic (non-motor symptoms, pre-diagnosis). Pons, medulla, cerebellum.
Figure 12.

Phase 2: perithalamic (motor symptoms, resulting in diagnosis). Basal ganglia, limbic system.
Figure 13.

Phase 3: suprathalamic (higher centres and later stages of disease.) Cortical regions.
Figure 14.

Figure 12

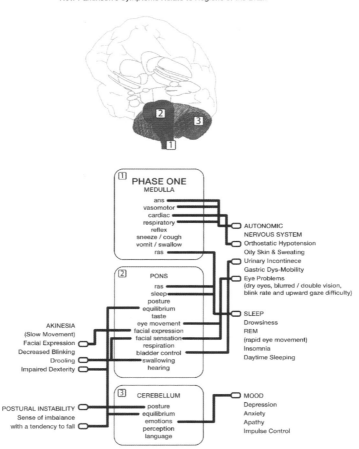

PHASE ONE
How Parkinson's Symptoms Relate to Regions of the Brain

116

Figure 13

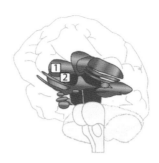

PHASE TWO
How Parkinson's Symptoms Relate to Regions of the Brain

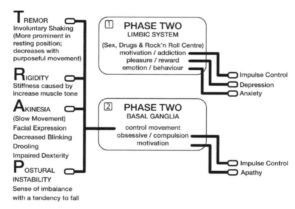

TREMOR
Involuntary Shaking
(More prominent in
resting position;
decreases with
purposeful movement)

RIGIDITY
Stiffness caused by
increase muscle tone

AKINESIA
(Slow Movement)
Facial Expression
Decreased Blinking
Drooling
Impaired Dexterity

POSTURAL
INSTABILITY
Sense of imbalance
with a tendency to fall

1. **PHASE TWO**
LIMBIC SYSTEM

(Sex, Drugs & Rock'n Roll Centre)
motivation / addiction
pleasure / reward
emotion / behaviour

Impulse Control
Depression
Anxiety

2. **PHASE TWO**
BASAL GANGLIA

control movement
obsessive / compulsion
motivation

Impulse Control
Apathy

Figure 14

PHASE THREE
How Parkinson's Symptoms Relate to Regions of the Brain

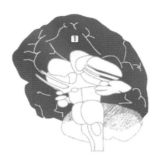

1 PHASE THREE
CEREBRAL CORTEX

Later Stages
Dementia
Cognition

Figure 15

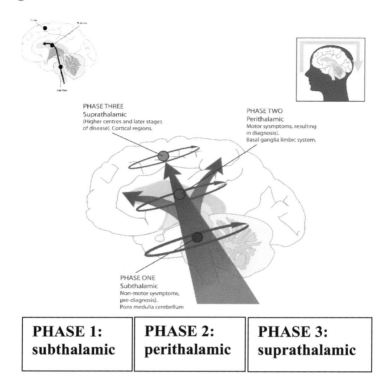

PHASE THREE
Suprathalamic
(Higher centres and later stages
of disease). Cortical regions.

PHASE TWO
Perithalamic
Motor sysmptoms, resulting
in diagnosis).
Basal ganglia limbic system.

PHASE ONE
Subthalamic
Non-motor sysmptoms,
pre-diagnosis).
Pons medulla cerebellum

PHASE 1: subthalamic	PHASE 2: perithalamic	PHASE 3: suprathalamic

What we have at present is an incomplete model, which focuses on the chemical dopamine and increasing motor function. Dopamine is manufactured in the pars compacta within the substantia nigra and this is currently thought to be where the problem lies. The reasons for, why and how this begins remains unexplained and is a matter for conjecture and debate. This present model has paid little or any attention to non-motor symptoms. The text here will, I hope, encourage changes in current thinking. It may even lead to alternative opinions and ideas.

The PPN

The pedunculopontine nucleus (PPN), as its name suggests, is in the posterior upper region of the pons. Arousal, attention, learning and reward are some of the functions involved, but more significantly, this particular part of the brain is involved in locomotion, limb movements and REM sleep. Recent studies suggest this area is mainly used for relaying sensory feedback signals to the cortex. However it was once thought to be an important part of initiating limb movement (i.e. motor).

A study involving deep brain stimulation on the PPN of patients suffering Parkinson's measured change in preparation and execution of movement[40]. Evidently, the PPN - when working with the basal ganglia - is an area of the brain involved in bringing about movement in the body. The results of this study showed it to be pro-kinetic and instrumental in maintaining posture and gait which are affected by Parkinson's.

This is further evidence that the pons is significant in Parkinson's in conjunction with conventional basal ganglia structures.

Others have also considered the Pedunculopontine nucleus (PPN) worthy of investigation. On the 7 June 2011, Mr. Alex Green delivered a lecture in Oxford entitled:

---

[40] See Tsang EW, Hamani C, Moro E, Mazzella F, Poon YY, Lozano AM, Chen R., *Involvement of the human pedunculopontine nucleus region in voluntary movements* as published in the journal: Neurology (vol 75, no.11), September 14, 2010 (Epub 2010 Aug 11)

Pedunculopontine nucleus stimulation for the treatment of drug resistant freezing and falls in Parkinson's Disease[41].

The PPN is part of the reticular activating system (RAS). The PPN projects axons to a wide range of brain regions, such as the lower brainstem, cerebellum, subthalamic nucleus, substantia nigra, pars compacta, globus pallidus internus, thalamus, basal forebrain, cerebral cortex, supplementary motor area, somatosensory and motor cortices.

Therefore, the PPN is of great importance in relation to PD. Along with other areas of the pons which send signals from the forebrain to the cerebellum, it has a role in sleep, generating the dreams of REM sleep. It also plays a part in respiration, regulating the change from inspiration to expiration. As well as all this, the pons has, as the diagram shows, roles in equilibrium, eye movement, facial expressions, facial sensation, posture, hearing, swallowing, bladder control and taste. It also receives inputs from other brain regions. I hope the reader can see the proposed relationship I make here between these regions of the brain and PD.

Motor and Movement Pathways

Ascending and descending pathways are important to understand but difficult to visualise. A diagram (**Figure 16**) is provided to assist instead of solely relying on descriptive terminology which can be confusing.

---

[41] See also: Thevathasan, Pogsyan, Hyam, Jenkinson, Foltynie, Limousin, Bogdanovic, Zrinzo, Green, Aziz and Brown, *Alpha oscillations in the pedunculopontine nucleus correlate with gait performance in Parkinsonism,* Brain Advance Access published January 9, 2012 (@ doi:10.1093/brain/awr315)

Figure 16

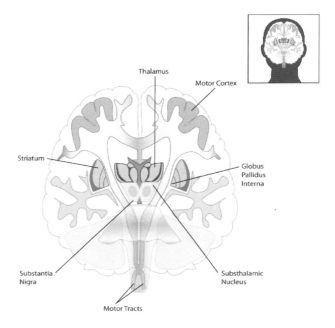

There are two tracts which relay sensory and motor information running up and down the spinal cord, brainstem, and basal ganglia to cortex. The sensory pathway passes information – let us say temperature or pain from your fingers - up the posterior (back) part of your spinal cord ultimately reaching a region called the somatosensory cortex. This then relays that information to the adjacent motor cortex. Signals then travel down the anterior (front) of the spinal cord instructing your muscles to remove your hand from the hot surface.

That is a greatly simplified version of these tracts. The regions through which these pathways can have a modulating effect on passing signals.

There are times when the brain overpowers instinct, allowing, in the long run, more advantageous actions. For instance, you may burn yourself whilst getting the Sunday roast out of the oven. A fast withdrawal reflex results in letting go of the hot dish leaving a broken plate and your dinner all over the kitchen floor. Alternatively, you may resist this *let go* instinct and keep a firm grip on the plate until it is safely placed on the table, burning yourself slightly, but happily saving the Sunday dinner.

Now we can use the above example to describe how the regions of the basal ganglia and the brain stem structures are of great importance in modulating movement. These areas of the brain are also known to be linked with movement disorders such as Huntington's and Parkinson's. However, as I see it, the brainstem structures may be more capable of this modulation than we currently understand. This modulation is not only on the motor output side, but is linked to the sensory input side and, if you look at the diagram, one can see the motor pathway clearly and in close proximity to the basal ganglia but also, more importantly, running through the brainstem region. A brainstem structure called the reticular formation is known to have this modulating effect on sensory and motor information and I feel this area needs greater investigation.

I believe the pons and perhaps the cerebellum have a contributing role in the modification of relayed signals. Conceptually, this will increase the complexity of the already intricate circuitry of the basal ganglia by adding extra circuits to the pre-existing model. Here, then, is an addition for the basis for our understanding of the movement disorder element we associate with Parkinson's.

123

One can now see the interrelationship of neurological structure and function and its importance in regard to Parkinson's symptoms. See diagram **Figure 11** which illustrates the structure/function model.

It can be seen that idiopathic PD symptoms follow a three-phased chronological progression in regions of the brain, stemming from the brainstem (with the non motor symptoms making diagnosis difficult) through to the mid brain where PD diagnosis is easier (due to more obvious motor symptoms and signs). Later, cortical symptoms (such as dementia) may or may not manifest themselves in the phase three area.

It is this base or brainstem region that will be the first affected from ischemic conditions from the vertebral artery. Then, degenerative changes follow the pathway of the vertebrobasilar arteries. So, from this view point, it can be seen that early treatment vantage point is possible. This will be explored further on. Before this, we must consider further evidence.

Chapter Ten

Supporting Evidence

Supporting Evidence

Now, I will further justify this hypothesis.

The brain uses 20% of the body's blood requirements but is only 2% of the body's mass. Therefore, the brain stem is a high consumer of blood and its contents. The carotid arteries supply blood and nutrients to the cerebral hemispheres which deal with the brain's higher functions, which are always in demand. The brain stem is supplied by the vertebral arteries.

The brain stem and especially the vertebral artery, in my view, are important to increase our understanding of neuro degenerative disorders. Some may argue, that the vertebral artery is of little consequence as the carotid arteries eventually join with the vertebral artery in the anastamosis of the circle of Willis and blood can pass from one artery to the next along the line of least resistance. In other words, there is a backflow or retrograde flow of blood from the carotid artery that would theoretically supply the brain stem via the basilar and vertebral arteries, as it can with subclavian steal syndrome if blockage occurs.

Those who see the vertebral artery as irrelevant to the problem of Parkinson's and perhaps other neurodegenerative disorders should be asking why there are two main arterial supplies to the brain in the first place. If the vertebral artery were that insignificant, evolution would surely have made it surplus to requirement. If there is a significant loss of blood normally supplied by the vertebral artery then this reduction must result in impaired function somewhere down the line.

As for degenerative changes narrowing the inner diameter of the carotids, there will likely be changes in the vertebrobasilar system at the same rate. The carotids I feel have a better chance of compensating for these degenerative changes due to their size and anatomical position.

However, the vertebrobasilar arteries are smaller and anatomically more constrained due to their location and pathway, so degenerative changes here will have greater consequences.

Using an analogy to UK plumbing, let us think of the vertebral artery as a 15mm pipe and the carotid artery as a 22mm pipe. Now, we can apply the same physics that are used for plumbing. There are three main elements to rate of flow: one is the hydraulic radius (size of pipe); the next is the friction coefficient (smoothness of pipe); then we have the pipe length (volume of fluid). The first two are important when looking at arterial flow as degenerative changes in the artery mean a reduced hydraulic radius and furring or clogging of the arteries will increase the friction coefficient thus increasing turbulence of flow. This means clogging of the smaller arteries, such as the vertebral, will require greater pressure to achieve the same rate of blood flow. Fluid viscosity may also be a factor influencing blood supply. Therefore, a smaller pipe means there will be a smaller supply of blood and nutrients to meet the brain's high-demanding requirements.

Judging by the approximate difference in artery size, we may assume that the vertebral artery supplies approximately one third of the brain's mass. The carotids, then, supply the remaining two-thirds. The difference between the vertebral artery diameter and the carotids is proportionate to the blood supplied to the brain (one third vertebral, two thirds carotids).

With the diameter of the vertebral artery reduced, some of the much needed blood will in theory come from the backflow of the carotid, I hear the reader proclaim. But, if there is reduction or obstruction in the blood flow to the vertebral arteries, especially in the basilar artery area (due to its position), the potential for backflow to the brain stem will be minimal.

Conversely, if occlusion occurs in the carotids, the vertebral artery has some potential to take over supplying blood to the rest of the brain, albeit in a limited capacity. So, in the first scenario (occluded vertebral arteries), there will be a lack of nutrients to the brainstem but not in the latter (occluded carotids) as the carotid artery has only just reached its destination (i.e. the brain). Backflow through the carotids will make little difference to blood and nutrients reaching the brainstem and can only occur if there is free flow through the arteries. Occlusion of any sort will limit the potential for backflow through, in this case, the vertebral artery.

To clarify, narrowed arteries result in reduced blood supply which in turn leads to neural dysfunction or cell death.

I would like to give an example here to demonstrate the importance of the vertebral artery for those that consider it insignificant and I apologise in advance for the macabre subject matter.

When an animal is slaughtered, consciousness may be maintained due to continued blood supply from the vertebral artery if this is not severed. This is the case with religious methods of slaughter such as Halal or Shechita. Studies have shown animals to be conscious up to 3 minutes after their carotids have been cut. In this way, scientists have linked blood supply to the brain with active consciousness[42]. We should not underestimate the significance of the vertebral artery and the role it has to play in supplying blood to the brainstem and the function the brainstem provides.

Having said all this, I am aware there will be some quick to dismiss my ideas. These may site a study in 2005 on extracranial blood flow in Parkinson's. The evaluation of a research team based at Afyon Kocatepe University in Turkey suggests that PD is 'not associated with a flow volume or velocity alteration of extra-cranial cerebral arteries.'[43] Given that intracranial blood supply is dependent on extra-cranial arteries, one may assume that blood flow is not, as I advocate, a significant factor in PD's pathology.

This 2005/6 study used 28 non-demented PD patients and 19 control subjects. The study aimed to disclose whether or not blood flow (or haemodynamic alteration) is a factor in PD.

This study however, did not go far enough to give any significant or reliable conclusion nor does it satisfactorily explain why a decrease in regional cerebral blood flow had been seen prior to their testing in relation to PD. It will remain a grey area until further extensive studies are

---

[42] See M,. Haluk Anil, *Religious Slaughter: A Current Controversial Animal Welfare Issue at* http://animalfrontiers.fass.org/content/2/3/64.full

[43] From abstract of: Haktanir A, Yaman M, Acar M, Gecici O, Demirel R, Albayrak R, Demirkirkan K; *Evaluation of extracranial blood flow in Parkinson disease*, Neurosci Lett. 2006 Jan 2;391(3):131-5. Epub 2005 Sep 23 (found: http://www.ncbi.nlm.nih.gov/pubmed/16183201)

carried out on larger patient numbers using more reliable diagnostic technology[44].

Other objections to my hypothesis may come from those who know that vertebrobasilar strokes tend to cause any of the following: headaches, nausea, sensory changes, visual defects or disturbances, speech disturbances, ataxia (i.e. walking and balance difficulties), vertigo, incontinence and drop attacks/blackouts. These symptoms do not match idiopathic PD symptoms. So, it would seem that an occlusion of the vertebral artery leads to symptoms which do not, at first hand, appear to correlate with the onset of Idiopathic Parkinson's or other neurodegenerative disorders such as I am arguing.

However, there is a difference between narrowing/occlusion and blockage. As I have said previously, strokes have a quicker onset and more significant impact whereas narrowing of smaller arteries will have a more insidious onset. Please take a moment to look again at the diagram that relates symptoms of PD with the functional areas of the brainstem, midbrain and limbic system. Here, you will see that the symptoms of Parkinson's - both motor and non-motor – bear a functional relationship to specific regions of the brain.

This objection is all well and good if we look at isolated areas of research and do not compare and contrast them with all other research on PD. This also assumes that we

---

[44] In their text, *Sampling and Sample Size Calculation,* Fox, Hunn and Mathers remind us: "From common sense, we see that the larger the sample is, the easier it is to be satisfied that it is representative of the population from which it is drawn" (p.13) @rds-eastmidlands.nihr.ac.uk/.../9-sampling-and-sample-size-calculation.ht...

[45] H Rafael, *Mesencephalic ischemia and Parkinson's disease Correspondence*, J Neurol Neurosurg Psychiatry 2004;75:511

all accept Parkinson's categorisation as a neurodegenerative disorder. Neurosurgeon, H Rafael does not. In commenting on a paper written by Y Abe on vascular impairment in the brains of Parkinson patients, Rafael states that Parkinson's disease has been 'wrongly classified'[45]. He even acknowledges his belief that Parkinson's disease begins in posterior perforating arteries as a consequence of the clogging of arteries or as he puts it 'atherosclerotic plaques located at the mouth of these arteries.'[46] This region, I feel, may be too specific. Also, consequences other than atherosclerotic plaques may be responsible for reduced blood flow in this area.

Y Abe and his team studied the brains of Parkinson's patients who did not have dementia and compared them to healthy subjects. According to the resulting paper, they 'confirmed that occipital hypo-perfusion is a common feature of PD patients without dementia.'[47] Therefore, these PD patients had reduced blood flow. One may argue that this has no significant relation. This, they may protest is irrelevant to the issue of PD pathogenesis. I believe otherwise and, on the contrary, Abe's conclusions reinforce my thinking. This study also has common ground with the findings of Dr Peter Jannetta who performed surgery on PD patients to relieve pressure on arteries resulting in diminishing PD symptoms[48].

So, strokes will result in damage to the brain. This is obvious but what about microvascular ischemia? The midbrain has long been identified as an area subject to deterioration, and is also a target area of the Parkinson's

---

[46] Ibid
[47] Y Abe et al, *Occipital hypoperfusion in Parkinson's disease without dementia: correlation to impaired cortical visual processing* As published in J Neurol Neurosurg Psychiatry 2003;**74**:419-422
[48] See Ref. 7

pathology. So, it is not at all unreasonable to suggest that vertebrobasilar microvascular ischemia (especially affecting the brainstem and later the midbrain) will eventually, though not immediately, instigate PD.

Additional supporting PD research looking at the influence blood supply has on the brain:

Heart health

There is another important factor which will play a part in adequate blood supply reaching the brain and this is cardiac output. Studies have made reference to this being a factor normally associated with dementia[49] but, with my proposed theory of slow vascular changes seen in Parkinson's, one can transpose the same link.

Dr Angela Jefferson surmised a link between decreased blood flow and brain atrophy. Atrophy is where the brain mass diminishes which occurs as the brain ages. It is more severely pronounced in Alzheimer's which is a sub category of dementia. Jefferson compared cardiac output to changes in brain structure. Poverty of blood flow provides fewer nutrients and less oxygen to the brain cells. Her study showed a correlation between heart and brain health[50].

It seems to me, then, that neurodegenerative diseases (especially those pertaining to the cerebral cortex associated with the dementia spectrum) are linked with

---

[49] In the Medscape Today (2012) article, *Cardiac Disease and Cognitive Impairment*, for instance, Laura HP Eggermont et al state: 'cardiac disease is associated with increased risk for cognitive impairment and dementia.' (see http://www.medscape.com/viewarticle/769847)
[50]See: http://www.emaxhealth.com/1506/reduced-heart-function-can-lead-brain-atrophy-dementia

vascular diseases. These could be either carotid artery specific or, as I have been suggesting with Parkinson's, vertebrobasilar artery specific and ultimately due to the consequence of neurovascular ischemia.

This is not in the same way as vascular dementia is conventionally viewed (sudden macro-vascular damage), but in alignment with the Evan's neurovascular hypothesis (slow ischemic micro-vascular changes) from mostly internal occlusion.

Exercise

Vigorous exercise can be seen as the silver bullet of most diseases today and seems to be increasing in popularity for treatment of neurodegenerative disorders. It has been known to be an effective rehabilitation technique for decades if not centuries now. More recent research has focused on why specific mechanisms may have a neuroprotective effect.

Dr J Eric Ahlskog writes about the difference exercise makes in the article *Does Vigorous Exercise Have Neuroprotective Effect in Parkinon's Disease?* The answer to his article's title is a resounding yes. Research shows that exercise provides protection from dopaminergic neurotoxins 'apparently mediated by neurotrophic factors'[51]. Mental processes are also improved and links to increased neuroplasticity, that remarkable ability and flexibility the brain has - on a cellular level - to adapt. This same study, found that non-activity (or, in the case of those animal 'models'

---

[51] See J. Eric Ahlskog, PhD, MD, *Does Exercise Have a Neuroprotective Effect in Parkinson Disease* in Neurology *July 19, 2011 77:288-294, Wolters Kluwer Health*

experimented on, 'immobilization') had the reverse effect. Significantly, humans' vulnerability to Parkinson's is decreased thanks to regular exercise during middle-age. Those PD patients who went on to exercise, were able to increase cognitive scores in tests but also their brain matter – more specifically, their cerebral grey matter and that this gain was proportionate to the amount of exercise they did. As a result of this study, practitioners involved in treating PD are advised to implement incremental fitness and exercise programmes for PD sufferers.

Exercise increases heart rate and volume of blood thus accelerating transport of nutrients and oxygen in optimal or plentiful amounts to any given target area, increasing the rate of cellular regeneration and restoring normal function. This dispenses with the need for any of these specific factors and neuroprotective mechanisms. All healthy cells require optimal levels of nutrients and a good supply is instrumental in cell regeneration.

Exercise, diet and healthy living (i.e. avoiding excessive alcohol, cigarette smoking and recreational drugs) in combination are seen as the natural 'cure-all'. Yet, despite people's increasing awareness, problems still exist. Some have difficulty motivating themselves for physical activity, despite knowing the benefits (especially those in their forties and above). In addition to this, some have problems with control over their diet and drug consumption. One could write an entire book on these subjects entitled: *Why we don't do what is good for us.*

Let us now look at contrasting additional research, which appears to illogically contradict healthy living and explain why unhealthy people, who smoke cigarettes, drink too much alcohol, are on medication for blood pressure and cholesterol, and drink coffee excessively, are actually less likely to get Parkinson's disease.

Smoking (Cigarettes and Marijuana)

Surprisingly, in recent times, it has been found that there are specific positive effects to cigarette (Smoker's Paradox) and marijuana smoking, especially helping those with neurological conditions. This is, of course, in addition to the many detrimental effects of smoking and marijuana. Here, we find that marijuana and nicotine have vasodilatory effects which facilitate blood flow to the brain[52]. Marijuana can have an effect on cardiac output by changes in heart rate and blood pressure as well as significant changes in regional cerebral blood flow. Brainstem vasodilation is an important protective factor in relation to the treatment of Parkinson's.

A study entitled *Enhancing Activity of Marijuana-Like Chemicals in Brain Helps Treat Parkinson's Disease* by Robert Malenka and Nancy Pritzker published in Nature (issue dated February 8, 2007) revealed that endocannabinoids in conjunction with the dopamine mimicking drug quinpirole proved effective in treating Parkinson type conditions in mice. The authors of the study claim this could lead to a new therapy for humans suffering Parkinson's. Endocannabinoids occur naturally in the brain and share similar characteristics to compounds found in marijuana. The mice treated were able to move freely after being in an immovable state. We have already discussed the vasodilatory effects of marijuana and its potential beneficial effects on Parkinson's disease. What

---

[52]Several studies such as: Toda & Okamura, 1991; Toda, 1975; Lee & Sarwinski, 1991; Lee *et al.*, 1996 show that nicotine causes vasodilation in cerebral arteries such as the basilar artery, middle cerebral artery and the circle of Willis in several animal species.

is interesting and new (as the researchers discovered) is that Dopamine combined with another drug - which slows enzymatic breakdown of endocannabinoids - appears to have an expediential effect (about 5-6 fold increase in motor activity). This drug combination modulates circuits in the striatum resulting in the normalisation of Parkinson's mice. As can be seen, this takes us beyond the territory of the substantia nigra which is in general thought to be the main area where Parkinson's is concerned. As I have been saying all along, changes in regional cerebral blood flow are significant and should be thoroughly investigated.

Similar studies on nicotine revealed a positive outcome. One possibility is that nicotine's action stimulates dopamine but this is uncertain. Smoking has even been recognised to help those suffering psychosis or schizophrenia. It has a biphasic effect (that is, to constrict, then to dilate) on the small arteries of the brain. Vasodilation is due to the effect nicotine has on nitrous oxide production. The vasoconstriction seems partially due to thromboxane. Work to develop drugs based on nicotine without the negative effects of smoking is underway and may be useful for future treatment and prevention of Parkinson's.

Alcohol

Picture a person, struggling to speak clearly, appearing lethargic and stumbling, having co-ordination difficulties and unable to pull their keys, wallet or phone from their pocket. Thinking of Parkinson's, one may consider this person to be suffering neurological symptoms. On the other hand, after reading the title 'Alcohol', you may very well jump to the conclusion the person is drunk. Adding location and context, one will come to an assumption far more quickly - a pub, for example, or, alternatively, a hospital. However, as appearances can be deceiving, you may be mistaken when you assume that the person you see struggling to stay on the pavement by a pub on a Friday evening is drunk when actually this person has neurological symptoms which resemble excessive drinking.

It is greatly surprising then that research as recent as 2013, shows that drinking beer, in particular, reduces the risk of Parkinson's. This revelation comes from a study involving no less than 300,000 people[53]. Specific alcoholic drinks were examined. Wine and spirits were found to make no significant difference. Specific reasons for this remain, as yet, elusive.

Indeed, though not specifically linked to PD, another study (involving 1,825 people aged 55 – 65) showed a tendency for those who drink alcohol to generally outlive those who do not, and this includes heavy drinkers[54]. Frontal Cortex journalist Jonah Lehrer suggests in his article, *Why Alcohol is Good for You*, that the reason for this is not so much in alcohol itself, as for the social contexts it facilitates, which induces production of good dopamine levels and other healthy chemicals in the brain[55]. When we think of how stress affects the body, we are on to another reason for the benefit of alcohol. Stress has been recognised as a major factor to a variety of life-threatening diseases and alcohol has the short term therapeutic effect of reducing stress levels.

---

[53] See Liu R, Guo X, Park Y, Wang J, Huang X, Hollenbeck A, Blair A, Chen H, *Alcohol Consumption, Types of Alcohol, and Parkinson's Disease* [@http://www.ncbi.nlm.nih.gov/pubmed/23840473]
[54] ibid
[55] See Jonah Lehrer, *Why Alcohol is Good for You*, Frontal Cortez wired science blog @ www.wired.com/.../2010/09/why-alcohol-is-good-for-you

Nevertheless, we must not simply take this as a licence to abandon ourselves to drink. There are, of course, many studies which highlight the negative effects of alcohol. Excessive drinking leads to heart disease, cancer and brain damage. Alcohol's toxic effect on the brain has been linked to various neurological conditions; it has even been suggested as a chemical cause for PD and these are in stark contrast to the recent 2013 studies that place alcohol in a more favourable light. If one is to take heed of these recent studies, excessive drinking is best avoided. Moderation is, as ever, recommended.

Caffeine

As with nicotine, caffeine has a vasodilatory effect. For some only, coffee will help prevent Parkinson's disease[56]. Coffee, also, has been shown to have some neuroprotective effect. There are negative side effects to caffeine use also, but again drugs are being designed to overcome them. Drug trials using caffeine have led researchers to conclude that there may be genetic factors involved as the drug's effectiveness works with only a quarter of patients (approximately).

Genetic

There is an ongoing debate as to whether genetic factors and/or the findings of alpha synuclein hold any significance. It is, for example, unclear whether autosomal dominant monogenic Parkinsonism is due to synuclein or LRRK-2 mutations. More likely there is a genetic predisposition towards those with young-onset Parkinson's. Obviously, genetics has a part to play in

---

[56] See article: *Gene Explains Coffee's Effects on Parkinson's* by Maggie Fox (http://blogs.reuters.com/search/journalist.php?edition=us&n=maggiefox&)

most pathology and there are now many genetic links to Parkinson's.

For this book to remain understandable I will avoid the complexity of genetics. Genetic and stem cell factors can be found easily in current mainstream research.

Placebo

The Placebo effect is when a patient's belief in treatment (often a pill) will influence how the body responds to illness. Its effect is so significant that it can, occasionally, have a greater effect than real medicine. This paradox has had researchers questioning how this phenomenon can be exploited for patient benefit.

One *un***orthodox** trialed treatment involves the placebo effect. Patients who participated in a Placebo Surgery Trial in 2004 reported an improved quality of life after receiving pseudo transplants of 'human neurons.'[57] Such treatment has interesting implications. Studies on this phenomenon indicate a 'mind-body connection' whereby a patient's belief in a particular type of treatment will influence how the body responds to the disease. The placebo effect is a well known phenomenon in the medical research profession. The difference here is the mode of treatment. Usually, placebo treatment is in the form of a pill. However, surgical placebo trials may raise an ethical eyebrow as surgery is invasive.

---

[57] See *Mind-Body Connection in Placebo Surgery Trial Studied by University of Denver Researcher* in *ScienceDaily* (April 8, 2004)

High Blood Pressure Medication

The key to modern day treatment of Parkinson's has been addressing the problem of dopamine. This has been dealt with by drugs that mimic neurotransmitters which, as we have seen, only have a short-term effectiveness. One way to advance such treatment would be to protect or rejuvenate existing brain neurons/regions together with the associated neurotransmitters.

A study conducted by Prof Surmeir at the US Northwestern University found in 2007 a substance able to protect brain cells[58]. It was isradipine, a drug that is classed as a calcium channel blocker and is primarily used to treat high blood pressure. This drug had the effect of protecting receptors in the brain and relieving the burden on neurotransmitters by channelling calcium ions which would otherwise prove problematic. Prof. Surmeier thought stress on neurons might explain why they die more rapidly as we age.

Prof. Surmeier serendipitously discovered, whilst working on a different problem, that neurons stop producing sodium and become more reliant on calcium to function. By using isradipine a calcium blocker, Prof. Surmeier discovered a way to force the neurons to start using sodium again.

The study showed great promise for the use of isradipine, a calcium channel blocker in the treatment of Parkinsons and was to be followed by another study involving 7,374 men and women over age 40 which was conducted in 2008 by Dr Christoph R Meier of Switzerland. Meier

---

[58] See: http://www.outsourcing-pharma.com/Preclinical-Research/Blood-pressure-drug-also-rejuvenates-brain-in-Parkinson-s

found evidence that high-blood pressure pills that are calcium channel blockers reduce the risk of Parkinson's disease by 23 percent[59]. For Meier, though, the explanation was elusive. More research is needed to discover why exactly this is so and to determine if this has any causal association to PD.

One other pertinent fact appeared to be that no other type of high blood pressure pill (such as beta blockers) worked to this effect.

Neurons use sodium when young and over-rely on calcium when old. Isradipine, as mentioned before, resulted in neurons using sodium again. If the brain could restore its youthful state, it would effectively reverse the problems of aging in the brain. So, it really is a question of age.

Incidentally, a group of Stanford University researchers in 2012 discovered that young blood rejuvenates the brain. The experiment was conducted on old mice which were injected with the blood of young mice. An anti-aging effect on the brain became apparent and the research signposts the way for future treatment on neurodegenerative diseases[60].

All these studies point a direction Parkinsonian treatment may go in the future. The reason this type of blood pressure pill benefits PD patients relates to my neurovascular hypothesis.

---

[59]See published article in the February 6, 2008, online issue of Neurology®, the medical journal of the American Academy of Neurology

[60] See article *By* Adam Clark Estes *of* The Atlantic Wire – *Thu, Oct 18, 2012 04:59 BST Young Blood Reverses the Signs of Aging*; found @ C:\Users\Connor\Desktop\Young Blood Reverses the Signs of Aging - Yahoo! Lifestyle UK.mht

Why, then, is it that high blood pressure pills which are not calcium channel blockers do not benefit PD sufferers? The answer could be, I feel, down to their effect on blood flow. Vasodilators work generally in two ways. Calcium channel blockers and nitrates work directly to relax the arteries.

The other method is through inhibition of vasoconstriction. In this method, ACE inhibitors block the activity of enzymes which stops angiotensin II, a powerful vasoconstrictor, from working.

Pills such as beta blockers work, as their name suggests, by blocking beta 2 receptors in the heart, slowing the heart down thus reducing blood pressure and flow. We now see a reason why some high-blood pressure tablets such as beta blockers do not help the treatment of PD as these slow blood flow.

Conversely, other research proposed Mitochondrial dysfunction, oxidative stress and inflammation to be significant factors in the advancement of Parkinson's Disease[61]. This research suggested that AT2 has no role in the development of PD. However, it is thought changes in AT2 receptors during the natural aging process might increase the risk of PD[62].

There is an interaction between angiotensin (AT2) and dopamine observed in the striatum, substantia nigra and renal cells. It was suggested that dopamine and angiotensin counter-regulate one another[63].

---

[61] See Marie-Odile Guimond and Nicole Gallo-Payet; *The Angiotensin II Type 2 Receptor in Brain Functions: An Update;* from International Journal of Hypertension Volume 2012 (2012), Article ID 351758, 18

[62] ibid

[63] Jose L Labandeira-Garcia, Jannette Rodriguez-Pallares, Ana I Rodríguez-

Some may infer from this that the decrease in dopamine brings about an increase in AT2. However, what if this actually works the other way round? An increase in angiotensin (such as in those with high blood pressure), reciprocally decreases dopamine levels leading to PD motor symptoms. Also, this complements my hypothesis as Angiotensin is a vasoconstrictor and, therefore, there will be a decrease in blood flow to the brain as well as the effects of reciprocally decreasing dopamine.

Other than this, the neurovascular hypothesis reasonably explains why calcium channel blockers work well for PD treatment and gives an alternative explanation to the findings in the various studies. I speculate cardiovascular medicine may play a key part in the future of medical treatment advancement of PD.

The relation between blood pressure pills and neuro-activity is still not fully understood. Perhaps there are reasons other than the effects calcium ions have on protecting receptors in the brain. Vasodilation is more likely to be the answer as increased blood supply to the brain would have a positive effect on brain chemistry. Indeed, this is what my hypothesis suggests.

Perez, Pablo Garrido-Gil, Begoña
Villar-Cheda, Rita Valenzuela, Maria J Guerra; *Brain angiotensin and dopaminergic degeneration:*
relevance to Parkinson's diseas; Am J Neurodegener Dis 2012;1(3):226-244www.AJND.us /ISSN:2165-591X/AJND1210003
http://www.ajnd.us/files/AJND1210003.pdf

Statins

In 2007, a Boston University research team found that particular types of statins significantly reduced the onset of Parkinson's and Altzeimer's[64].

Statins are used to reduce cholesterol by impeding plaque accumulation in the arteries of the brain. However, the researchers claim that only simvastatin gives the worthwhile effect of cutting Alzheimer's and Parkinson's by 50% and that the other two statins tested (atorvastatin and lovastatin) did not fare so well, suggesting an additional effect particular to simvastatin. This additional effect may have been anti-inflammatory or due to a change in the rate of beta-amyloid secretion but this was far from certain. Possibly, simvastatin is simply more effective at reducing cholesterol than the other statins studied.

Although the researchers have asked the question why statins should help Parkinson's and Alzheimer's, are they missing the obvious? I think the neurovascular concepts (as explained in the previous chapter) again answers why such a powerful statin should make a difference.

Statins reduce atherosclerotic plaques inside the blood vessel which accumulate on the arterial wall. These atherthosclerotic ('fatty') plaques lead to cardiovascular disease. A reduction in these plaques will increase cardiovascular blood flow as there will be less obstruction within the arteries.

---

[64] Specifically, researchers from Boston University School of Medicine (BUSM); see the Future Pundit article, *Simvastatin Cuts Alzheimers And Parkinsons By Half*, at **http://www.futurepundit.com/archives/004399.html**

Koh KK in a Cardiovascular Research article published in 2000, stated that the 'beneficial effects of statins on clinical events may involve non-lipid mechanisms that modify endothelial function, smooth muscle cells, and monocyte-macrophage: vasomotor function, inflammatory responses, and plaque stability.'[65] In other words, statins are effective in helping reduce resistance of blood flow through arteries by various mechanisms[66].

So, statins do more than just reduce fatty plaques (that tend to stick to the arterial wall); they also increase the lumen diameter (i.e. the internal diameter of a blood vessel). We begin to see the promise of statin vasodilation with regard to blood supply to the brain and how this may be used in future treatment of PD.

Again, this vasodilatory consideration further complements my neurovascular proposition.

In searching for evidence on vasodilatory effects of statins, we find that that there are more effective and less effective statins. As previously mentioned, the Boston University research team, having tested a number of statins, claimed Simvastatin significantly reduced the onset of PD and dementia. Although Atorvastin did not have quite as powerful an effect in this regard it nevertheless was found to have a notable effect whereas Lovastatin was not found to have any significant effect of this kind at all.

---

[65] See Koh KK. *Effects of statins on vascular wall: vasomotor function, inflammation, and plaque stability*, Cardiovasc Res. 2000 Sep;47(4):648-57

[66] See also Mukai Y, Shimokawa H, Matoba T, Hiroki J, Kunihiro I, Fujiki T, Takeshita A., *Acute vasodilator effects of HMG-CoA reductase inhibitors: involvement of PI3-kinase/Akt pathway and Kv channels*, J Cardiovasc Pharmacol 2003 Jul;42(1):118-24.

Looking at research into the vasodilatory effects of statins, we find that 'statins act as coronary vasodilators.' Specifically, 'Simvastatin, cerivastatin and atorvastatin but not lovastatin induced vasodilation.'[67]

Let us latch on to the statement that statins act as coronary vasodilatory which specifies the heart. We may then assume that there will be the same vasodilatory effect on all arteries including the brain.

This lack of vasodilatory effect in lovostatin is exactly the link we are looking for and explains why lovostatin was not effective where simvastatin was very effective in treatment of PD. This explains why Lovastatin showed no beneficial effect for PD patients. We still have questions for investigation; chiefly:

-   What level of vasodilatory effect might Simvastatin have over atorvastatin?

This question poses a grey area in the research. The Boston research in 2007 overlooks the difference in vasodilation between sinvestatin and atorvostatin. There would have to be something in addition to the vasodilatory effect of simvestatin. However, one can not easily dismiss this vasodilatory factor as atorvostatin still had a beneficial effect. Furthermore, we have already explored much to favour vasodilation as far as fighting off neurodegenerative disorders is concerned. Nevertheless, I

[67] See Lorkowska B, Chlopicki S Prostaglandins Leukot Essent Fatty Acids., *Statins as coronary vasodilators in isolated bovine coronary arteries--* involvement of PGI2 and NO. 2005 Feb;72(2):133-8.

.

speculate that atorvastatin will be found the lesser agent in vasodilation than simvestatin. It may indeed be that Simvastatin has the most powerful vasodilatory effect as well as a de-clogging effect that the other statins do not possess.

Researchers appear not to have considered vasodilation as an important factor in explaining simvestatin's wonderful effect. Instead, they suggest the explanation may lie in an anti-inflammatory effect or a beta-amyloid secretion from the drug.

Currently, there is some controversy on statins because there are fears that statins are over-prescribed[68] and have side-effects in healthy people. There is even a study conducted in 2007 suggesting that statins may increase the risk of PD[69]. This seems paradoxical, especially in light of the research we have looked at that advocates the benefits of statins for PD sufferers. Nevertheless, British Heart Foundation's Professor Peter Weissberg, commented on this particular 2007 study insisting: "There is no evidence to suggest statins cause Parkinson's disease."[70]

With so much hype on simvestatin, one may wonder why such studies are started in the first place and indeed who decides on what drug is to be tested. The question of who initiates such studies is always linked with motivation and motivation may distort whatever is found. Some might

---

[68] See the November 2010 Live Science article by Jospeh Brownstein, *Statins May Be Over-prescribed* at http://www.livescience.com/8981-study-statins-prescribed.html.

[69] See the Telegraph article by Nic Flemming (dated 15 Jan 2007) at http://www.telegraph.co.uk/news/uknews/1539534/Scientist-fears-statins-link-to-Parkinsons.html

[70] ibid

say that sound research should be free from vested interest and/or conflicts of interest, including any relationships with people or organizations that could inappropriately influence a study. Incidentally, UK medical research often favours the Cochrane Review[71] as the place to go for unbiased evidence-based medicine as it considers research from other organisations. Unfortunately, nothing relevant can presently be found regarding this area of statins and Parkinson's.

Even so, there is enough indication from the studies mentioned above that vasodilatory effects make a positive impact on those suffering PD.

These findings are very significant in supporting my hypothesis. I speculate future treatment will involve use of a poly-pill, part statin, part vasodilator and part dopamine which will improve symptoms and, more importantly, work towards a cure having a neuro-regenerative effect.

Conclusion

In conclusion, increased blood flow to the brain (vaso-dilation with increased cardiac output) has a positive effect on brain health and Parkinson's disease, and the vertebral artery is, for me, of paramount importance. There are several possible explanations as to why the vertebral artery may be compromised in the first instance. The consequences this will have - in terms of deficiency of oxygen and other nutrients transported to the brainstem - are, at present, speculative in relation to Parkinson's symptoms and signs.

---

[71] See *The Cochrane Collaboration* at http://www.cochrane.org/cochrane-reviews

The pons, medulla and cerebellum are usually viewed independently. To study them in isolation risks limited thinking. These brainstem structures should be regarded as working together with the basal ganglia region and the limbic system (especially the nucleus accumbens).

Collectively the brain stem, basal ganglia and limbic system are significant areas of the brain; certainly, they also should not be treated separately in regard to Parkinson's (see Tri-phase model). Together they process, modulate, inhibit or stimulate ascending (sensory) or descending (motor) information. They are all, along with the cortex, in certain ways, communicating and are perhaps orchestrating discovered and undiscovered interrelated pathways.

I consider the substantia nigra and the basal ganglia region a small part of a more complex circuitry which has yet to be discovered or understood fully. The brainstem should be explored further for a relationship with the basal ganglia and limbic system. I suspect there is an important brainstem interconnection that has, until now, not been found and, as I have so often mentioned, the cerebellum, medulla and especially the pons play an important role. We should also bear mind how these regions of the brain work within the wider context of the complete human body.

We must not forget the overall framework within which these parts operate. If we do, we may easily lose sight of the problem at hand and miss the opportunity of being able to fix it.
It seems that research focussed on discovering specific mechanisms often neglects the reasons why brain cells are degenerating in the first place. Looking at entire systems

instead of sub-systems brings into play unwanted complex variables, especially in humans, but it might be prudent to have a glance back once in a while or we risk missing the overall picture.

Keeping complete biological systems in mind is bound to bring us to a closer understanding of Parkinson's as well as many other diseases.

Chapter Eleven

Testing the Theory

Proposals for Testing the Theory

Validating hypotheses and theoretical work requires practical testing. Having explained my neurovascular hypothesis, it is now appropriate to convey my recommendations on how my ideas can be investigated. As my work hinges on the vascular system, it is pertinent to describe the vertebral and basilar arteries. From there, I will proceed to outline my proposals for practical research.

The origin of the vertebral arteries is from the sub-clavian arteries, on both sides (bilaterally). They then enter the transverse process at the level of the 6th cervical vertebrae (C6) moving superiorly, through the transverse foramen until C1. Then they cross the posterior arch of the atlas before entering the foramen magnum. The two vertebral arteries join inside the skull to form the basilar artery - the main blood supply to the brain stem - at the base of the medulla oblongata. They later connect to the circle of Willis where it joins the carotids.

Figure 16

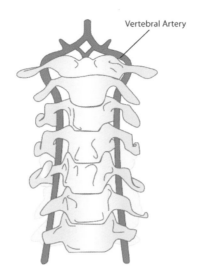

Vertebral Artery

I would start testing by x-raying the diameter of the vertebral artery foramina. This artery has a tortuous route through foramina in six cervical vertebrae. This is an unfortunate design fault or anomaly to which the term *critical zone* could be applied as it is in other areas of the body such as the avascular region of the supraspinatus tendon (1cm from its insertion)[72] as well as the blood supply to the spinal cord around T4 to T9[73].

These x-rays would determine whether or not degenerative or post traumatic changes are reducing one

---

[72] Age and position dependent (i.e. above 40 years: adduction and distraction increases the avascularity)

[73] The blood supply to the spinal cord is shown to be the least rich, and the spinal canal narrowest, from the T.4 to approximately the T.9 vertebral level. This is in the region of the mid-thoracic spine, between the shoulder blades, T9 being the area near to the bra-strap.

or more of the foramina diameter in the neck. Such a reduction is likely to compress the vertebral artery resulting in a poverty of oxygen and nutrients to the brain stem and thalamic structures. Data of this kind would reveal whether a significant reduction in blood supply leads to regional ischemia of the brain and so result in disorders such as PD.

Secondly, it would be prudent to view the internal diameter of the vertebral artery by modern day scanning techniques (such as PET[74], fMRI[75]) and make an assessment of regional cerebral blood flow together with cardiac output. Cross-referencing these data, observing any correlation with Parkinson's patients, may further support the theory.

Also, a study similar to Dr Jefferson's could be implemented to see if there is a link between heart health and Parkinson's. Cardiac output is significant and may indeed be part of the cause as opposed to being just a symptom. It could be that low blood pressure in Parkinson's is a consequence of vasomotor changes in the brain stem. Control of the heart (ANS) would then diminish hence the low blood pressure. Alternatively, it may be that PD is exacerbated by reduced blood flow to the brain from low blood pressure/cardiac output. In this scenario, ischemia is likely to starve regions in the brain of oxygen as described in the previous chapter.

Human trials and animal studies also need to be conducted. I will be seeking opportunities to work with

---

[74] PET scans measure and track the flow of blood using labelled radioactive chemicals in the brain.

[75] fRMI stands for functional Magnetic Resonance Imaging. This involves placing a patient inside a large and powerful magnet. The scan displays those areas of the brain with a greater supply of oxygen. It is cheaper and more sensitive than a PET scan and does not use radioactivity.

research groups in the near future to progress this work so that improved treatment can be implemented for those suffering Parkinson's and I will explain ways in which this can be achieved below. Nevertheless, I think it is important to share this message now, as further research and acceptance of new concepts takes considerable time.

Chapter Twelve

Beyond 21st Century Treatment

Beyond 21ˢᵗ Century Treatment

It is my view that integrating two separate fields of medicine (vascular and neurological) will give us a more pragmatic perspective to bring about a greater treatment effectiveness of neurodegenerative diseases. Future treatment of PD is likely to involve the use of neurotransmitters, namely dopamine, in combination with vasodilatory drugs and consider statins. This would reduce the current dose of dopamine, thus reducing side-effects, and enhance performance concurrently. These drugs combined in the form of a poly pill perhaps, would be easy to implement as they have already been trialled and are in current use for treatment of other diseases. This may bring about a regenerative and neuroprotective effect if early diagnosis is attained. One can see a clear, obtainable route to effective treatment resulting in either prevention or a cure.

Given that the problem is a deficiency of blood supply to certain areas of the brain, it follows that these blood vessels need to be widened to restore the required blood flow and normal brain function. One way of enabling this is by use of vasodilatory medication.

Medication in the form of vasodilators may be implemented quickly, safely (excepting some restrictions[76]) and cheaply. These vasodilators could also be used in conjunction with statins then fMRI testing can be used to assess any change in cerebral blood flow via the vertebral artery.

---

[76] Caution is needed for patients with certain medical conditions such as being at risk of brain haemorrhage or raised inter-cranial pressure. This may be contraindicated.

Vasodilators work generally in two ways. Calcium channel blockers and nitrates work directly to relax the arteries. The other is through inhibition of vasoconstrictors. In this method, ACE inhibitors block the activity of enzymes which stops angiotensin II, a powerful vasoconstrictor, from working.

Unfortunately, there are side-effects to these types of drugs, most of which are mild. Using them will lower a patient's blood pressure which can lead to headaches, dizziness and fainting (etc.). The prescription of vasodilators comes with a caution for individuals who suffer unstable blood pressure and this may be a problem as Parkinson's patients may have problems with low blood pressure. This, no doubt, can be rectified or modified in some way. Perhaps statins only or in conjunction with dopamine medication would be more advisable.

Research has recently been dropped by some pharmaceutical companies as neurodegenerative disorders have become less appealing and research funding has been awarded to more high profile areas of research such as cancer. Government spending on research now prioritizes food security and bio-technology/energy and shows a neglect of research into brain related disorders. UK cuts alone in the next five years amount to a figure of around 20 million pounds, resulting in the closure of pharmaceutical and university research centres. This has affected my local area with 2,500 job losses in one company alone.

One would have second thoughts, as a young researcher, pursuing a career in neuroscience in the UK. David Nutt, a professor of neuropsychopharmacology said 'There is now virtually no neuroscience being done by pharmaceutical companies in Britain,' and described the future of neuroscience in the UK as 'extremely bleak.'[77] It was reported in February 2011 that many surviving research facilities will relocate to China. This reflects the current economic crisis and sadly demonstrates that money drives scientific advancement; thus, lack of funding slows the progression of innovative medical development.

Professor Barbara Sahakian, Professor of Clinical Neuropsychology at the University of Cambridge said that if pharmaceutical companies withdrew from cancer research 'the outcry would be enormous.' She also implied that there is a stigma surrounding mental illness (another projected increasing area of medicine in need of funding) and that this has had a detrimental effect[78] on funding.

Funding is an issue plaguing scientific research that will most probably be controversial for as long as there is scientific research. How much should be spent and on what exactly? Criticism has been made against funding the Human Brain Project that aims to virtually recreate the human brain using a supercomputer. Other, perhaps more worthwhile projects have been deprived or even aborted as a result. We are, after all, talking of one billion euros awarded as a European research prize, a vast amount of money even in this day and age.

---

[77] See article: *Neuroscientists attack cuts to brain research funding* by Harriet Bailey published 15 February 2011
(http://www.newsciencejournalism.net/index.php?/news_articles/view/neuros cientists_attack_cuts_to_brain_research_funding/)

[78] Ibid

Henry Markram is the director of the Human Brain Project and defends it by mentioning the Human Genome Project. Despite the fact that this project did not live up to its many promises, scientific advancement was made all the same[79]. Markham describes it as 'a mechanistic approach that one change may bring about multiple other changes. No one knows the results that could come of it, which may lead to something unknown becoming known.'

The Human Brain Project is about having an artificial brain to simulate all kinds of research into neurology. In theory, this would dispense with the need to use actual human brains for neurological research.

The New Scientist reports 'a growing demand' for human brain samples in the interests of research into neurodegenerative diseases 'as animal models aren't mirroring the disease too well.'[80] David Dexter is the director of a bank of such 'sample' brains and says: 'The holy grail is to develop neuroprotection'. He goes on to explain: 'The convolutions of the brains are like fingerprints - no two brains are the same. If you look at 'normal' brains that come into the bank, about 15% of them aren't normal. They've got early stages of neurodegenerative disease.'[81]

Currently, Research teams with limited funding may request tissue from Dexter's 'brain bank' and receive free samples. This is in huge contrast to the substantial sum granted to the Human Brain Project.

---

[79] See Griggs, Jessica; *One Minute With Henry Markram* in *New Scientist* no.2903; 9 February 2013; page 29
[80] See Hooper, Rowan; *Our Brain in Their Hands* in *New Scientist* no.2903; 9 February 2013; page 10
[81] ibid

Although animal test subjects do not always make ideal models for human neurodegenerative disease, they are still used for this purpose nonetheless. A recent model showed great promise. Mice with prion disease[82], considered 'the best animal representation of human neurodegenerative disorders'[83], were given a compound which restored healthy protein production in their brains, thus halting the disease.

A major problem with neurodegenerative disease is with malformed (or misfolded) protein. We have identified this earlier when looking at Braak's alpha-synuclein Lewy bodies.

Advances in this area were made at the University of Leicester's toxicology unit UK. A Medical Research Council (MRC) team led by Professor Giovanna Mallucci established that build up of these ill-formed proteins results in the cessation of the production of new proteins. This is due to a natural defence mechanism in cells that is trying to compensate for the overabundance of misfolded proteins. Malluchi's team introduced a compound which prevented this 'switching off' protein production. The results were so promising that media presenting their findings announced a breakthrough in neurodegenerative research. The MRC's project has been hailed as 'an exciting and historic moment in medical research'[84]. A cure is, perhaps, no less than 20 years away as some

---

[82] CJD in humans is a type of prion disease as is bovine spongiform in encephalopathy (BSE, better known as Mad Cow Disease). Prion disease affects the structure of the brain and is currently untreatable and fatal.
[83] See http://www2.le.ac.uk/offices/press/press-releases/2013/october/medical-research-council for the article: *Medical Research Council scientists discover compound that arrests neurodegeneration in mice*; issued by MRC on Wednesday 9 October 2013
[84] See Robert H Olley, *Halting neurodegeneration in mice – a possible cure for Alzheimer's?*, October 10th 2013 [http://www.science20.com/R.H.Olley]

announced[85]. Indeed, the normal behaviour in the test subjects (mice) was restored and memory loss prevented. However, as a side effect, the pancreas of each mouse was damaged leading to diabetes and such weight loss of at least 20% that meant the mice had top be destroyed (in accord to Home Office regulations) preventing further study. Despite seeing 'the disease stop dead in its tracks', Mallucci acknowledges we are 'still a long way from a usable drug in humans' as 'this compound has serious side effects.'[86] Nevertheless, the study, as MRC's Professor Hugh Perry said, 'might eventually aid the development of drugs to treat people suffering from dementias and other devastating neurodegenerative diseases.'[87]

Journalist Robert Olley identifies the MRC study as the 'first time that any form of neurodegeneration has been completely halted so, it is a significant landmark'[88]. Incidentally, the MRC invests taxpayers' money in medical research and given the impact Mallucci's study, demonstrates public funding being put to good use. One may also assume that the amount of money involved here does not reach the staggering billion euros given to the Human Brain Project.

My own Neurovascular study has not deprived any neuroscience project as it has not been funded. Though, to explore my hypothesis with rigour and ascertain its promise will most certainly require this.

Hopefully, the text here will renew pharmaceutical interest in the medicinal treatment of neurodegenerative disorders such as Parkinson's and this, in turn, will

---

[85] *MRC study - BBC news website.*
[86] See note 82
[87] See note 82
[88] See note 83

readdress the balance of funding in UK research. Pharmaceutical companies have a vested interest with this type of research which I hope they can exploit/develop for the greater good of the patient. For the time being, researchers will pursue Dexter's 'holy grail' of neuroprotection with their slices of free brain tissue.

Vasodilation must be considered to be one way forward in achieving neuroprotection. Increasing the supply of oxygen and nutrients to the brain is crucial for protecting aging brains. It is likely, as mentioned earlier, lack of oxygen and nutrients from poor blood supply leads to cellular impairment or damage at the level of the DNA which in turn results in defective protein synthesis and the malformation or misfolding of proteins such as, in the MRC study on mice with prion disease (mentioned above). So, for PD the protein is alpha-synuclein, in Huntington's it's the Huntington protein and in Alzheimer's its amyloid and tau proteins. We know there are other mechanisms to this process but this is a possibility worth looking into.

Effective treatment depends on achieving an early diagnosis. If this could be attained and the patient is treated within the window of opportunity (Phase 1) regenerative results are more likely. After Phase 2 in our model, the treatment is less likely to have these desired regenerative effects as brain damage will more likely than not be irreversible. Therefore early diagnosis is essential.

The problem we have currently is, that, this early diagnosis of Parkinson's disease is difficult to achieve. Patients who show symptoms of the early stages could be screened. If reduced blood flow through their vertebrobasilar artery is detected, we then have a diagnostic indicator and treatment may be administered early. Therefore, the more advanced symptoms of Parkinson's diseases can be avoided altogether; prevention being better than cure.

Routine scans could be performed on anyone (aged, say, 50 plus) in much the same way breast scans are used. Preventative early diagnostic screens would highlight one's propensity to the onset of idiopathic Parkinson's and similar disorders through detection of reduced regional blood flow to the brain; thus preventative advice/medication could be administered early, again halting the process of neurodegeneration.

Cardiac output as previously mentioned is an important factor in blood reaching the brainstem. Blood flow through small arteries and cardiac output are difficult to measure. Nevertheless, assuming we can obtain reliable figures for both these values, I propose the following equations based on the results of the vertebral artery flow test:

$$V \times C = D$$

> Where V is the figure representing the blood flow through the vertebrobasilar artery; C, the Cardiac output; and D = the diagnostic figure used to determine if there is a propensity for onset of Parkinson's symptoms. Figures V and C could be given values 1-10 (1 being poor blood flow and 10 meaning excellent blood flow). Patients will vary with regard to V and C. Thus, a safe numerical figure for both V and C being, say, 5, D's value of around 25 would be deemed within safe parameters and a favorable result[89]. A result significantly below 25 would warrant further investigation.

---

[89] I have given this idea to serve as a mere starting point. The function of the equation and its accepted parameters may be modified.

A further consideration is cost. This cost of screening for early prevention of Parkinson would be outweighed by the money saved that would otherwise be spent on the long term care, treatment and hospitalization of these patients. Government spending and cuts are an ongoing concern affecting the medical profession.

Recently, the government's decision to cut funding to Parkinson's nurses[90] resulted in a study into long term cost effects. Savings now are likely to bring about future costs. Indeed, it is projected that there will be significant future expense as patients end up being admitted more frequently to hospitals. Money in the long term would be lost rather than saved by cutting funding to Parkinson's nurses.

Exploiting the Blood Brain Barrier and Visual and Auditory Cues

The blood brain barrier makes delivering certain chemicals to particular areas of the brain problematic. This is because it acts as a neuroprotector by keeping out toxic substances and selectively letting beneficial substances through. Unfortunately, it is not so discerning where therapeutic pharmaceutical substances are concerned, meaning that it will block a substance that would benefit damaged areas of the brain. However, future medicine may exploit modern technology and science such as nanotechnology (using loaded nanoparticles) or vaso-active substances to deliver drugs to target areas of the brain such as the pons, medulla or, as convention would have it, the substantia nigra where they are in deficit. Nanotechnology may also be useful in the

---

[90] See http://www.parkinsons.org.uk

diagnoses of Parkinson's as it is in other brain pathologies such as tumors.

Visual and auditory cues as previously mentioned exploit a phenomenon which benefits patients greatly. The mechanism of this phenomenon could be vascular based. However, it is more likely neurologically mediated. Either way, at the time of writing, it is unknown as to how this works.

In the Meantime

Until such a time that better treatment options become available, it is best to keep active if it is still physically (or neurologically) possible because, as in the Nun's study, you *either use it or lose it*. Safe options with probably minimal and limited effects are already currently used in the treatment of Parkinson's. These include exercise and relaxation techniques such as meditation and nutrition. All will have beneficial effects due in some part to regional and global vasodilation.

Exercise for PD patients[91]

We have already established the importance of exercise and this can never be overstated. It has been proven an effective therapy and likely to be preventative in most pathologies, reducing the risk of, cancer (colon 50%, breast 20%), heart disease and stroke (35%) and many other diseases including Parkinson's. Any type of physical exercise a person enjoys will yield results; it is not restricted to yoga and Pilates. Enjoyment is crucial

---

[91] See Appendix for list of books and websites for specific recommended exercises.

and better results are achieved when a person has fun and is performed with a social group, friends or trainer.

This is an area I would like to expand upon, perhaps, in another edition as exercise can bring great benefit, empowering the sufferer and giving them back some control over their movement, especially in the early phase of this disease. There are countless benefits of exercise on overall health, including enhanced mood, physiological improvements, positive biochemical and neurotransmitter effects as well as neural reprogramming and rehabilitation.

To keep things simple, sensible physical exercise is one of the best ways to slow progression of degenerative changes to the brain and body.

Two modes of exercise commonly used for PD patients are passive and active movement. Passive exercise involves a practitioner, carer or helper who manipulates limbs and encourages slow gentle movements. These include a large range of joint-movements and muscle stretching. Active exercise is where the patient self-directs and induces movement to help maintain muscle size, strength, tone, co-ordination, speed and joint range of motion. This is extremely helpful and has greater overall benefit than that of passive movement; however, a combination of these two is best.

The strength of large muscle groups can be important in maintaining controlled coordinated smooth movement. Combined contraction of the glutes, quads and hamstrings, with simple awareness of breathing and posture can be used for movements such as sitting slowly with controlled descent onto a chair. I use this example, as I have seen many patients who fall into a chair rather than actually sit. This is because they lack the strength in their thighs or feel unmotivated to exercise the muscles required to sit down. In the latter case, the muscles lose strength due to disuse and this often becomes habit. Actually getting up from the chair becomes even more of a struggle. Focussing on using these muscles and making these simple controlled movements will help to regain strength and ensure these basic everyday movements, we often take for granted, become easier.

Regular practice of physical exercise is vital and should begin with an incremental program of slow repetitive and rhythmic movements. Balance based exercises are recommended and developing new strategies for walking, standing and gait training.

Another problem to deal with is muscle freezing. Sometimes, touching a patient with muscle freezing is enough to break the freeze. The effort of self-induced movement when one feels the onset of muscle freezing is perhaps more useful as this is an independent action and independence is vital. This may begin, again, with simple rhythmic movements.

A carer or practitioner will not always be at hand and, usually, a patient will not want to become totally dependent on someone else being there. Some, lacking motivation due to depression, are in danger of becoming practitioner or medication dependent and this is neither good for the patient or their families. However, in advanced stages this may not be wholly avoided.

We know that patients often find tasks normally taken for granted problematic. These can be better tackled by breaking down the task into smaller, separate step-by-step tasks. Taking up hobbies and even maintaining existing ones is also recommended.

Finally, physical exercise alongside listening to music, singing and even humming a good tune is very much recommended. The practice of deep breathing is also beneficial. Research has shown all this to help alleviate anxiety, gain control over tremor, speech and everyday movements.

Chapter Thirteen

Ongoing Studies

Ongoing Studies

Questions to be Addressed

- What are the interactive mechanisms (i.e. chemical model and electrical/neural pathways) between the limbic system, basal ganglia and brainstem? Can new models be proposed?
- Can new evidence of this interconnection between limbic, brainstem and basal ganglia be obtained?
- How do neural circuits in the brainstem modulate neural activity in Parkinson's?
- What are the consequences of vertebral artery ischemia on brainstem function in relation to Parkinson's symptoms?
- How will vertebral artery ischemia effect modulation of neural circuits between limbic, basal ganglia and brainstem?

In Closing

In introducing and advocating a new hypothesis based on functional neuroanatomy, we see the possibility of a breakthrough in medical science on Parkinson's. Beginning by describing Parkinson's disease and outlining theories and research undertaken from James Parkinson's *Essay on the Shaking Palsy* through to the present day, we evaluate modern thinking on PD treatment and find it inadequate.

Clearly, there is a need for a new approach on the subject as well as a better way to treat those afflicted with this condition. I have presented and justified the neurovascular hypothesis also giving clear suggestions on how treatment may be conducted in the future. Here may be a long-term solution to problems with present treatment which may also be applied to other neurodegenerative diseases.

In presenting the neurovascular hypothesis, I am well aware that it has yet to meet the approval of those in the scientific community who are already engaged in research on Parkinson's and neurodegenerative diseases, so I am naturally curious to see how this will be appraised.

One may dismiss this work as it was neither instigated nor supported by some prestigious institution. I, however, see some advantages. Creative, independent thinking could have been compromised and I may have ended up working on something entirely unoriginal instead. Persuasion by others also moves one away from originality.

I am convinced that micro-vascular insufficiency and the pathogenesis of idiopathic PD are strongly associated, as well as many other neurodegenerative diseases, especially Lewy body dementia which is closely related. That said, it may not be solely responsible in all cases. Other factors may inevitably be involved and pathogenesis will be determined by a combination of circumstances. Nevertheless, even if this is the case to a degree with PD, I am confident vascular deficiency is the predominant problem. Knowing this is key to solving many neurodegenerative disorders including PD.

Now is the time for all medical practitioners who are involved in the treatment of PD to completely re-evaluate current theories. So far, this causative hypothesis of a vascular pathogenesis is theoretical. Further research is required to put this to the test and enable effective application of these ideas.

This hypothesis is in its infancy and I would like to test and fully explore all the ideas proposed here. At present, experimentation and testing is required so that it may mature into a fully validated theory. Research into this area will need funding and setting up. I am seeking opportunities to work with other experts in this field so that this hypothesis can be further investigated.

I am keen to hear from anyone able to give me feedback, especially those whom are actively involved in PD research. I appeal to others to join me in collaborative future research to explore and fully develop my hypothesis.

My hope is that this book will give sufferers and their families hope that there are people out there still searching for answers.

THE END

About the Author

Christopher Evans has been a clinician for almost 20 years working from his private practice in Kent. He also runs a neuro-rehabilitation consultancy. Occasionally, he works as specialist provider for rehabilitation following road traffic injuries.

From 1994-1999, Christopher undertook a full-time UK University validated course, graduating with around 10,000 hours of study and over 1000 hours of clinical supervised practice. Since then, he has worked tens of thousands of clinical hours. More recently, he completed post-graduate studies at University and in the last 10 years has run several practices locally in Kent but has also worked abroad.

In 2000 – 2001, he worked with professional dance group Spirit of the Dance on their European tour for one year (Germany, Belgium, Holland, Poland, and Denmark). During 2002, he treated international UK athletes at their warm weather camp in California and in Spain. Closer to home, he treated the local Rugby Club in 2005-6. In 2008, he was once again abroad, working at the European Veteran Championships in Slovenia, treating international UK athletes.

Christopher's patients are an eclectic mix of people including professional singers, musicians, dancers, athletes, and medical professionals including those suffering neurological symptoms.

He has been a member of several councils/associations and is currently a senior associate member of the Royal Society of Medicine London UK.

His background training prepared him for the research needed for this book, which included 5 years of human anatomy, physiology, orthopaedics, neuroanatomy, clinical neurology and neural science etc. Also, a part of this training included writing a 10,000 word dissertation on the physiological mechanisms of stress and how this manifests in humans. When investigating PD (in common with stress), he found most of the research dated back to the 1950's. He enjoyed studying the effects of stress on the brain and was influenced and intrigued by subjects such as post traumatic stress disorder. He worked with a number of PD patients and this was later to start his journey into PD research.

Christopher finds the human body and brain fascinating. "There is a lot more known about the brain now, than when I was a student," he says, "and it is easier now to access this information". He committed himself to investigating PD in the hope of finding something that would alleviate the suffering from this terrible affliction.

Early in his career he noticed that something was either missing or had been overlooked in the material he had read on PD. This stuck with him until the time was right and his curiosity led him to explore the research further. There is now plenty of material on PD but Christopher found that it had not progressed very far in the last 50 years. What is out there is inconclusive and variable. He noticed that this variability of results could be explained by his emergent hypothesis.

One of the key principles in his training is that tissue-repair needs an adequate and plentiful blood supply. It occurred to him that blood supply to the brain has been, for the most part, overlooked in the study and treatment of neurodegenerative disorders. Although a link has been made between cardio-vascular problems and strokes in relationship to neurodegenerative disorders, studies looking at micro-vascular changes and the anatomical position of the vertebral artery were somehow missing. He spent years searching for a positive correlation between blood flow to the brain and neurodegeneration. Then, in later research papers, this connection started to show up.

For more information on rehabilitation consultancy and free giveaways, visit the website enquiry section:-
www.parkinsonsdisease-trapped.co.uk

Please remember to leave your review on Amazon.

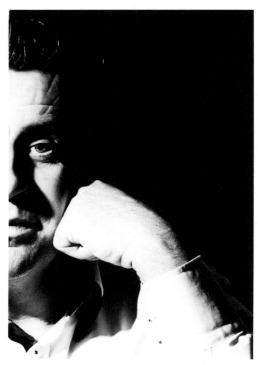

Glossary

adrenaline: a hormone secreted by the adrenal medulla of the adrenal gland above the kidney. Secreted during stress response. Elevates heart rate.

akathisia: inability to remain still. Restlessness. May be caused by reaction to neuroleptic medication.

akinesia: loss of motor control resulting in the inability to move voluntarily.

alpha synuclein: abnormal human protein found in the brain.

alpha-synucleinopathy: as above; commonly found in elderly patient suffering form a neurodegenerative disease.

Alzheimer's disease: neurodegenerative disease. Characteristic symptoms include memory loss, emotional instability and progressive impairment of mental capacity.

amantadine: anti-Parkinson drug; also anti-viral

amygdala: part of the limbic system; brain area involved with emotions such as fear and anger.

angiotensin II: octapeptide substance which constricts arteries; can increase blood presure.

antidepressants and antipsychotics: drugs used to treat depression and psychosis.

Arterio-sclerosis: reduction of the inner diameter of the artery (lumen) leading to reduced blood flow and degenerative vascular disease.

Autonomic disturbances: changes in the autonomic nervous system.

Autonomic Nervous System (ANS): controls involuntary action (non-conscious); made up of the sympathetic (speeds up heart/repiratory rate) and parasympathetic (slows rate down) nerves.

autosomal dominant monogenic Parkinsonism: forms of genetic Susceptibility to Parkinson's.

avascular region: area of reduced blood flow

basal ganglia: collection of brain nuclei involved in motor function or movement

bio-markers: substances used as indicators for particular conditions

bradykinesia: slowness of movement.

brain stem/brainstem: base of the brain; continuous with the spinal cord; includes pons, medulla and cerebellum.

cannabinoids: group of chemical compounds found in the drug cannabis.

carbidopa: Parkinsonian drug used in conjunction with levedopa.

Cardiac output: the force and the rate of heart contraction.

carotid arteries: largest arteries supplying the brain with blood

catecholamine: naturally occuring compounds that operate as hormones or neurotransmitters.

cerebellum: part of the brain involved in balance and co-ordination; located at the base of the brain (posterior/inferior)

cerebral artery: arteries supplying the cerebral hemispheres

cerebral haemorrhage: bleeding in the brain which can lead to stroke.

cerebral peduncle: large bundle of nerve fibres in the brain.

cervical vertebrae: bones of the neck.

chronic traumatic encephalopathy (CTE): sub-concussive and concussive trauma leading to neurodegenerative condition; normally linked with sports involving head injuries.

circle of willis: joining of several arteries in the brain near the pituritary gland

Comtan (Entacapone): Parkinsonian drug used in conjunction with dopamine-mimicking drug (such as levedopa)

cranial nerves: 12 pairs of nerves in the brain serving speech, taste, hearing, sight and smell

Deep Brain Stimulation: surgery involving electrical implants that stimulate dysfunctional areas of the brain.

dementia: loss of mental capacity involving memory, speech, emotions and decision making/problem solving; cognitive degeneration.

Diuretics: make you urinate more easily; usually in the form of a substance which affects the kidneys

dopamine: substance that helps regulate movement and emotion when produced in the brain

Dopamine Agonists: substance which assists the effect of dopamine

Dopamine dysregulation syndrome: disorder developed in Parkinson patients who become so addicted to their medication that they take more than the prescribed amount; an irregularity in the brain's reward system resulting from lengthy dopamine-replacement therapy; symptoms include excessive gambling, sexual behaviour, irrational repetive behaviour (punding) and eating.

dopaminergic neurons: nerves that manufacture dopamine found in the mid brain

dorsal motor nucleus: cell bodies that form the basis of the dorsal vagal nerve. Speeds up certain vital organs and slows others (eg. heart rate)

dyskinesia: slowness of movement with difficulty initiating movement.

Dystonia: involuntary muscle spasm.

endocannabinoids: naturally occuring substances within the body which are neuromodulatory lipids (i.e. fats that can either increase or decrease nerve impulses) having similar effect to cannabis.

entacapone: drug used to help dopamine mimicking drugs such as L-dopa to cross the blood brain barrier.

fMRI Functional Magnetic Resonance Imaging; type of diagnostic scan

foramen magnum: a large hole at the base of the scull through which the spinal cord passes.

glutamate: a salt that is excitatory in the central nervous system.

GABA: Gamma Amino Buteric Acid; inhibitory in the central nervous system; has calmining effect.

Halal: what is acceptable food (and preparation of) by islamic law. Slaughtering animals for food includes cutting the carotid arteries and hanging the animal upside down.

Huntington's disease: a disease of the mid brain or striatum which leads to the inability to control excessive or abnormal movement.

hyperhidrosis: increased sweating

Hypersexuality: increased sexual desire and/or activity

hypersomnolence: excessive or daytime sleeping

hypokinesia: reduced
movement

Hypotension: reduced
blodd pressure

ischemia: lack of blood
supply

iTrem: device designed
to detect tremor

kinesia paradoxa:
phenomenon
whereby a person
seemingly unable to
move suddenly,
stimulated by certain
conditions acquires
the ability to move
normally

levadopa: dopamine
mimicking drug

Lewy bodies: abnormal
protein found in the
brain and used in the
diagnosis of
Parkinon's and
dementia

limbic system: area of
the brain asociated
with emotion,

memory, basic drives
such as sex and
hunger. Homeostaic
mechanisms reside
here also. Located in
the midbrain.

locus coeruleus: part of
the pons; regulates
chemicals in response
to stress and panic

marijuana:
controversial drug
(from the canabis
plant) used
recreationally and
processed for other
medication. Active
chemical compound
it Tetra Hydra
Chloride (THC)

medulla oblongata:
situated at base of
the brain below the
pons. Controls
automatic functions
such as breathing
and heart rate.

Monoamine agonist:
class of anti-
depresent drug

motor accessory nerve: cranial nerve 11 (CN XI). Innervates the trapezius and sternocleidomastoid muscles.

MRI:
Magnetic Resonance Imaging scan

nanotechnology: involves manipulation of material on an atomic or molecular scale with a wide range of application including medical science.

nasal olfactory epithelium: a specialised skin tissue found in nose cavity that detects odours

neocortex: outer layer(s) of the cerebral hemispheres and part of the cerebral cortex engaged in higher functions such as conscious thought, reasoning, language,

motor commands and sensory perception.

neuroplasticity: ability of the brain to create new neural connections allowing it to adapt and change.

neuroprotective effect: the ability of any chemical to protect the nervous system against degenerative diseases
Neuropsychiatric symptoms: psychiatric symptoms found in neurodegenerative disorders.

neuropsychopharmacol ogy: combines neuroscience and psychopharmacology (study of how drugs effect the mind and brain).

neurotrophic factor: secreted protein that is involved in nerve growth in the brain.

Also called: Brain Derived Neurotrophic Factor (BDNF)

nicotine alkaloid chemical found in the tobacco plant and the substance to which smokers become addicted to. Also used in inecticides.

nigrostriatal axons: interconnecting nerve cells.

nucleus accumbens: part of the brain responsible for reward, addiction and motivation

olfactory: relating to the sense of smell

olfactory bulb: bulblike part of the brain where the olfactory nerves begin.

pars compacta: part of the substantia nigra that contains dark pigmented melanin cells.

pathogenesis: origin and development of a disease

Pathological gambling: impulse control disorder can be due to brain dysfunction.

pedunculopontine: located in the brain stem below the substantia nigra. Believed to be involved in initiation and modulation of movement as well as gait.

Peripheral oedema: swelling of extremities.

PET: Positron Emission Tomography; scanning that enables a 3 D image to be produced.

placebo: substance having no pharmaceutical properties but which may nevertheless bring about a positive pschological effect on the patient to which it is administered.

pons: part of the brain stem consisting of a group of nerve fibres connecting the cerebrum, midbrain and the medulla.

Postural (orthostatic) hypotension: the feeling of diziness and fainting when moving from a sitting of lying position to upright or standing due to a drop in blood pressure reducing blood to the brain.

Punding: repetitive and ritualistic behaviour involving pointless tasks such as touching and sorting objects. Usually this is a side effect of amphetamine drugs but also a symptom of Parkinson's and other brain disorders.

raphe nuclei: nuclei cluster situated in the brain stem; mainly functions to release seratonin to other parts of the brain

rasagiline: pharmaceutical monotherapy used in the early stages of Parkinson's; works by inhibitting the breakdown of dopamine.

REM sleep: a stage of sleep whereby Rapid Eye Movement occurs

selegiline: as with resagiline, this is an irreversible drug used to treat demetia and depression also used in the early stageParkinson's.

Shechita: jewish ritualistic slaughter of mammals and birds involving the cutting of carotid arteries, the trachea and esophagus, allowing the blood to drain.

sialorrhoea: excessive production of saliva

Sinemet: combination (Carbidopa and Levodopa) drug used in the treatment of Parkinson's

somatosensory cortex: outer lateral part of the brain involved in processing sensory information such as light, touch, pressure and pain.

stem cells: self-replicating cells that are able to transform themselves into more specialised cells. Now, in stem cell research and therapies, stem cells are artificially grown in a laboratory.

subclavian arteries, 35

substantia nigra: (black substance) region of the brain involved in producing dopamine

subthalamus: located below the thalamus; multiple functions

supraspinatus tendon: a tendon situated just above the spine of the scapulae

thromboxane: compound in the blood that facilitates blood clotting and constricts blood vessels.

Tourette's syndrome: severe neurological disorder identified by facial tics and obsene utterences as well repetive and involunatary movements.

transverse foramen: holes in the transverse process of six cervical vertebrae through which the vertebral artery passes.

tumors: an abnormal, uncontrolled growth of a group of cells.

ubiquitin: small protein found in most tissues

vagus nerve: 10th cranial nerve controlling the autonomic nervous system (things such as regulation of breathing, heart rate and bowel function); has both motor and sensory parts.

vascular Parkinson's: sudden onset of Parkinson's symptons due to stroke or vascular complications.

ventral pallidum: located in basal ganglia; involved in emotions, motivation and behaviour

ventral tegmental: A group of neurons located in the mid brain involved in cognition, motivation and addiction; also intense emotions relating to love and pschiatric disorders.

vertebral artery: an artery which provides blood to the brain via the brain stem.

vertebrobasilar system: the joining of the vertebral arteries and the basilar artery in the area of the brain stem or cranial base.

Index

Bibliography

Books

Halliday, Barker & Rowe (editors), *Non-Dopamine Lesions in Parkinson's Disease*, Oxford University Press, 2011

Anthony H.V. Schapira (ed.), *Parkinson's Disease*, Oxford Neurology Library, Oxford University Press 2010

Geofrey Leader and Lucille Leader, *Parkinson's Disease: Reducing Symptoms with Nutrition and Drugs*, Denor Press (2nd edition) 2009

Richard Secklin, *Parkinson's Disease: Looking Down The Barrel*, Nettfit Publishing 2010

Edwards, Quinn & Bhatia, *Parkinson's Disease and Other Movement Disorders* (Oxford Specialist Handbooks in Neurology) Oxford University Press 2008

Richard Secklin, *Marijuana for Parkinson's Disease: Cannabis Research & the Miracle Plant for Parkinson's*, CreateSpace Independent Publishing Platform 2012

Geofrey Leader and Lucille Leader, *Parkinson's Disease Dopamine Metabolism, Applied Metabolism and Nutrition*, Denor Press 2009

Kevin Lockett, *Move It!: An Exercise and Movement Guide for People with Parkinson's Disease*, Langdon Street Press; 1 edition 2009

Serge Przedborski, *Parkinson's Disease*, Cold Spring Harbor Laboratory Press 2012

Charles Tugwell, *Parkinson's Disease in Focus*, Pharmaceutical Press; 1 edition 2007

Journal Articles

Jefferson, Michael, *James Parkinson: A Medical History*, The British Medical Journal, 9 June 1973

Kaminsky, T. A., Dudgeon, B. J., Billingsley, F. F., Mitchell, P. H., & Weghorst, S. J. (2007). Virtual cues and functional mobility of people with Parkinson's disease: A single-subject pilot study. Journal of Rehabilitation Research & Development, 44(3)

Dopanimergic Neurons by Chinta and Anderson in The International Journal of Biochemistry and Cell Biology, May 2005

Tsang EW, Hamani C, Moro E, Mazzella F, Poon YY, Lozano AM, Chen R., *Involvement of the human pedunculopontine nucleus region in voluntary movements* as published in the journal: Neurology (vol 75, no.11), September 14, 2010

Lipton, Peter, *Ischemic Cell Death in Brain Neurons* in Physiological Review Vol. 79, No. 4, October 1999 (Printed in the USA)

J. Eric Ahlskog, PhD, MD, *Does Exercise Have a Neuroprotective Effect in Parkinson Disease* in Neurology *July 19, 2011 77:288-294, Wolters Kluwer Health*

Mind-Body Connection in Placebo Surgery Trial Studied by University of Denver Researcher in *ScienceDaily* (April 8, 2004)

T Yasui & Mkominyana; *Accessory middle cerebral artery and moyamoya disease*; Neurol Neurosurg Psychiatry *2001;71:129-130 doi:10.1136/jnnp.71.1.129*

Shen-Yang Lim, MBBS, FRACP; Susan H. Fox, PhD, MRCP; Anthony E. Lang, MD, FRCPC; *Overview of the Extranigral Aspects of Parkinson Disease;* Archives of Neurology *2009;66(2):167-172*

H Rafael, *Mesencephalic ischemia and Parkinson's disease Correspondence,* J Neurol Neurosurg Psychiatry 2004;75:511

Y Abe et al, *Occipital hypoperfusion in Parkinson's disease without dementia: correlation to impaired cortical visual processing* As published in J Neurol Neurosurg Psychiatry 2003

See J. Eric Ahlskog, PhD, MD, *Does Exercise Have a Neuroprotective Effect in Parkinson Disease* in Neurology *July 19, 2011 77:288-294, Wolters Kluwer Health*

Mind-Body Connection in Placebo Surgery Trial Studied by University of Denver Researcher in *ScienceDaily* (April 8, 2004)

Hinkle JL, Bowman L. "Neuroprotection for ischemic stroke". *J Neurosci Nurs* **35** (2) April 2003

Web Sites

http://www.parkinsons.org.uk

http://www.gladstone.ucsf.edu/gladstone/site/kreitzer/

http://www.youtube.com/watch?v=Nn3NYhnqGzY

http://www.healthstudies.umn.edu/nunstudy/faq.jsp

http://www.neurology.org/content/70/13/1042

http://www.emaxhealth.com/1506/reduced-heart-function-can-lead-brain-atrophy-dementia

http://blogs.reuters.com/search/journalist.php?edition=us&n=maggiefox&

http://www.newsciencejournalism.net/index.php?/news_articles/view/neuroscientists_attack_cuts_to_brain_research_funding/)

http://www.worldhealth.net/news/brain-blood-vessel-blockages-may-contribute-parkin/

http://www.cks.nhs.uk/parkinsons_disease

http://www.shef.ac.uk/news/nr/1772-1.174113

http://www.ncbi.nlm.nih.gov/pubmed for :

1. Parkinsonism Relat Disord. 2010 Feb;16(2):79-84. Epub 2009 Oct 28; *A timeline for Parkinson's disease* by Hawkes CH, Del Tredici K, Braak H.

2. Neurol Neurochir Pol. 2005 Sep-Oct;39(5):380-8; *Sleep disturbances in Parkinson's disease* by Boczarska-Jedynak M, Opala G.

3. Zh Nevropatol Psikhiatr Im S S Korsakova. 1977;77(1):51-5; *Characteristics of regional cerebral circulation in parkinsonism patients according the 133Xe clearance findings* by Man'kovskii NB, Vanishtok AB, Lizogub VG.

http://www.case.edu/med/epidbio/mphp439/Health_Care_Costs.htm (for: Georgia Zachopoulos, *Current Trends in Health Care Costs*)

http://faculty.washington.edu/chudler/aging.html (Neuroscience for Kids)

http://opdc.medsci.ox.ac.uk/

http://pdrecovery.org/index.htm

http://www.alzscot.org/pages/index.htm (for *Alzheimer's Disease: a Detective Story* by Professor Claude Wischik)

http://www.medicalnewstoday.com (for *An Early Step In Parkinson's Disease: Problems With Mitochondria* by Quinn Eastman) http://www.lewybodyjournal.org/whatlbdis.html   (for: *What Lewy Body Disease Is* from The Lewy Body Journal)

http://www.gladstone.ucsf.edu/gladstone/site/gind/

http://www.medicinenet.com/script/main/hp.asp

http://www.wellsphere.com/detailedSearch.s?keyword=Brain+Blood+Vessel+Blockages+May+Contribute+to+Parkinson%E2%80%99s+Disease+&x=33&y=11

http://www.emaxhealth.com/1506/reduced-heart-function-can-lead-brain-atrophy-dementia   (for heart function leading to brain atrophy)

http://blogs.reuters.com/search/journalist.php?edition=us&n=maggiefox& (for *Coffee's Effects on Parkinson's* by Maggie Fox)

http://www.newsciencejournalism.net/index.php?/news_articles/view/neuroscientists_attack_cuts_to_brain_research_funding/ (for: *Neuroscientists attack cuts to brain research funding* by Harriet Bailey published 15 February 2011)

30806161R00116

Made in the USA
Lexington, KY
18 March 2014